Supple Workout

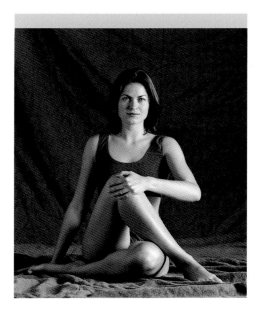

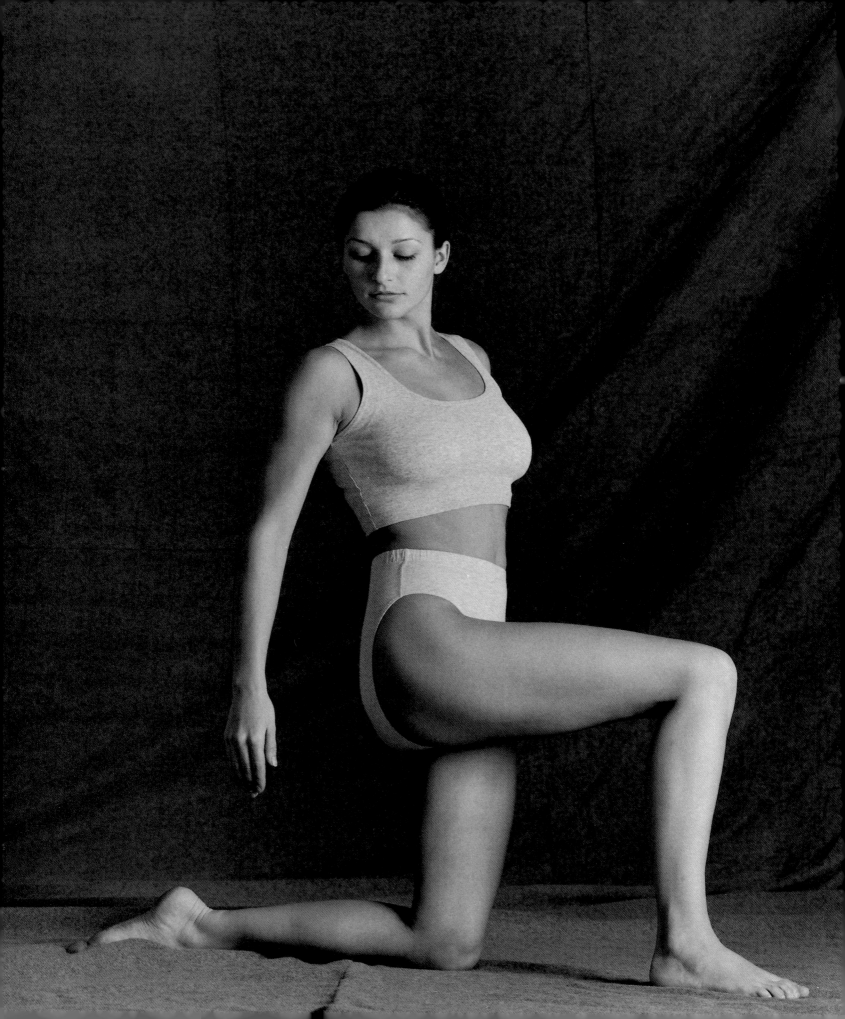

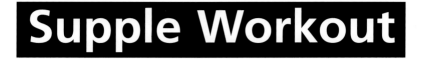

Supple Workout

Stretching for
Health and Flexibility

Lorna Lee Malcolm

Mark Bender

Photography by Antonia Deutsch

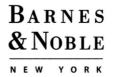

BARNES
& NOBLE

NEW YORK

Supple Workout
Lorna Lee Malcolm and Mark Bender

This edition published by Barnes & Noble, Inc.,
by arrangement with Duncan Baird Publishers

2001 Barnes & Noble Books

Conceived, created, and designed by
Duncan Baird Publishers Ltd.
Sixth Floor, Castle House
75–76 Wells Street
London W1T 3QH

Material from this book was first published in
the United States in 1996 by Macmillan in two
separate volumes from *The Supple Workout*
series: *Hips and Thighs* and *Abs and Back*.

Designers: Sue Bush, Gail Jones
Assistant Designer: Suzanne Tuhrim
Editor: Stephanie Driver
Assistant Editors: Georgina Harris,
    James Hodgson
Commissioned photography: Antonia Deutsch

M 10 9 8 7 6 5 4 3 2

ISBN: 0-7607-2358-3

Typeset in Frutiger
Color reproduction by Bright Arts, Hong Kong
Printed in Singapore by Imago

Publisher's note
The exercises in this book are intended for
healthy people who want to be fitter. However,
exercise under inappropriate circumstances can
be harmful, and even fit, healthy people can
injure themselves. The publisher, the authors,
and the photographer cannot accept any
responsibility for any injuries or damage
incurred as a result of using this book.

Contents

Introduction

Each body is unique. We all have different strengths and weaknesses, but all too often we fail to recognize our strengths and how useful these are in realizing the full potential of our body – this book shows us how to make the most of our body, with a toning program for more energy and confidence in ourselves.

For many of us with a modern, sedentary lifestyle, the hips and thighs are trouble-spots. But getting rid of the cellulite is not difficult. The first section of this book provides easy and enjoyable targeted exercises, that, combined with a healthy diet, will soon lead to a more toned and attractive body.

The second section focuses on your abs and back. The exercises lead not only to better appearance, as you stand straighter and your midriff is firmer, but a great sense of well-being, as you breathe deeply and feel the strength of your new, more dynamic body.

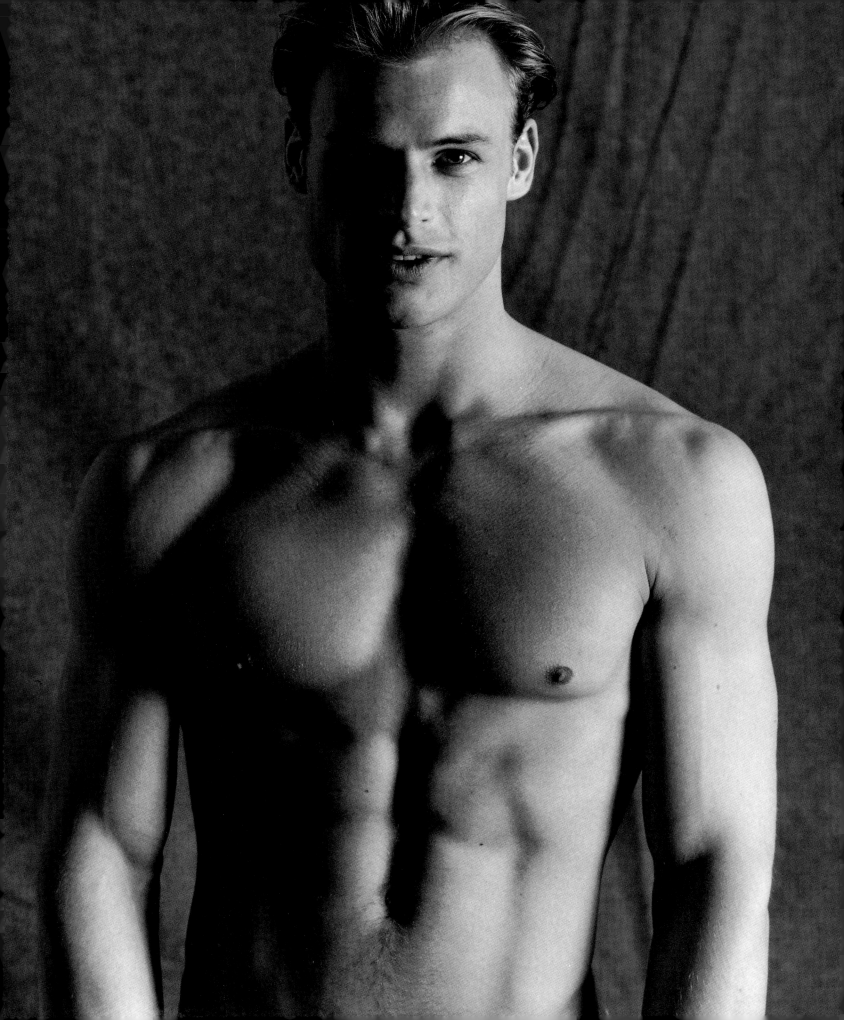

Getting started:
how to use this book

The exercises in this book are designed so that they do not require a major time commitment and can be adapted for your own schedule. You do not need any special equipment or clothing. Exercise should be safe and effective, but it should also be fun. Don't let your workouts become a chore. Exercise with friends, play music, vary your format.

When you are working from the Hips and Thighs section, use the following tips: for support, choose a chair that is sturdy and a good height, so you can hold the back of it comfortably, without bending or tilting. You can also enhance the exercises with weights. If you do not have hand weights, try holding cans of beans or tomatoes. Water bottles are even better – you can fill them with sand, rice, or whatever is to hand. Start with the bottles half-full, gradually adding weight.

When you move on to the Abs and Back section, bear in mind that success will be quicker if you integrate the Core Exercises with some of the exercises from the Total Body Workout section.

Before each session, do a posture check:
- Center your weight over both feet.
- Stand tall without locking your knees.
- Have your hips in a neutral position, neither too far forward nor back.
- Pull in your abdominals and lengthen your spine. Imagine that your back and abdominal muscles are strong and solid, like a metal belt around your waist, so you can stabilize yourself from within, maintaining good posture and body alignment. Whenever you see the words "stabilize your torso" in this book, think of this metal belt.
- Lift your chest up and press your shoulders back and down to maximize lung capacity.
- Hold your neck long and aligned with your spine, and ease your head back so your chin does not protrude.

The exercises in this book are safe if you follow the instructions correctly. However, if you have persistent lower back pain, consult your physician immediately. If you have severe spinal problems, it is best to consult your physical therapist or your physician before beginning any exercise program.

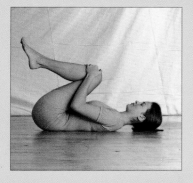

Warm-ups, pages 10–23
Before you begin to exercise, you should spend a few minutes warming up in order to get your muscles and joints moving freely, lessening the chance of injury. Similarly, you should devote time to the cool-down, gradually stretching the muscles you have worked and taking time to relax.

Hips and Thighs

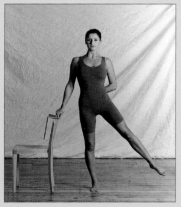

Core exercises, pages 38–55
These are the essential exercises for your hips and thighs. Organized by muscle group, they include both stretches and strength moves. To tone your hip-and-thigh area, you should try to do a selection of exercises from this section every other day.

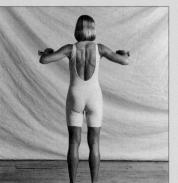

Total body workout, pages 56–71
These exercises covering the rest of the body complement the core exercises, so you can work toward overall health and fitness.

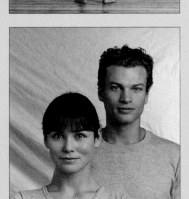

Routines, pages 72–81
In order to save time and keep yourself interested, you can combine exercises, developing a comprehensive workout covering your entire body. This section demonstrates key exercise combinations, giving you guidelines on how to devise your own.

Abs and Back

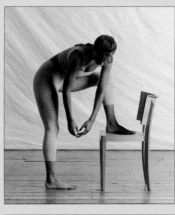

Core exercises, pages 96–117
Focusing on the abdominals and the back, these exercises will stretch and strengthen the muscles of your torso, helping you to develop a more vibrant and upright appearance and a healthier spine.

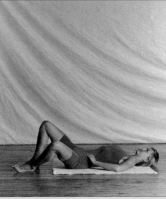

Total body workout, pages 118–131
These exercises are designed to increase the stability of your trunk and pelvis by working the muscles of your lower back, your abdominals, and your buttocks. Stronger muscles in the trunk and the pelvis will help the body to move more efficiently, lessening strain on the spine.

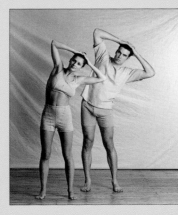

Routines, pages 132–141
It is easy to fit exercise into any lifestyle. Here are two examples of routines tailored for specific circumstances. Pause Gymnastics are exercises designed to be done regularly when you are working at a desk, in order to avoid strain in your back and arms. The Home Energizer exercises are perfect for people who do not play sports but want some simple but dynamic exercises to do at home.

Warm-ups

Warm-up exercises create several responses in your body. In general, they make you more mentally alert and bodily aware. More specifically, they will gently mobilize your joints, lubricating them and preparing them for activity. Your respiration will increase, so there is more oxygen available for your working muscles. Your heart rate will also increase, speeding the movement of oxygen-carrying blood around your body. Your nervous system becomes more sensitive during a warm-up, so nerve impulses or messages are sent from brain to muscle more rapidly.

The best time to work on gentle stretching to improve your flexibility is during your cool-down, when your body is warm. At the same time, slower movements will bring your heart rate, body temperature, and respiration gradually back to a normal level.

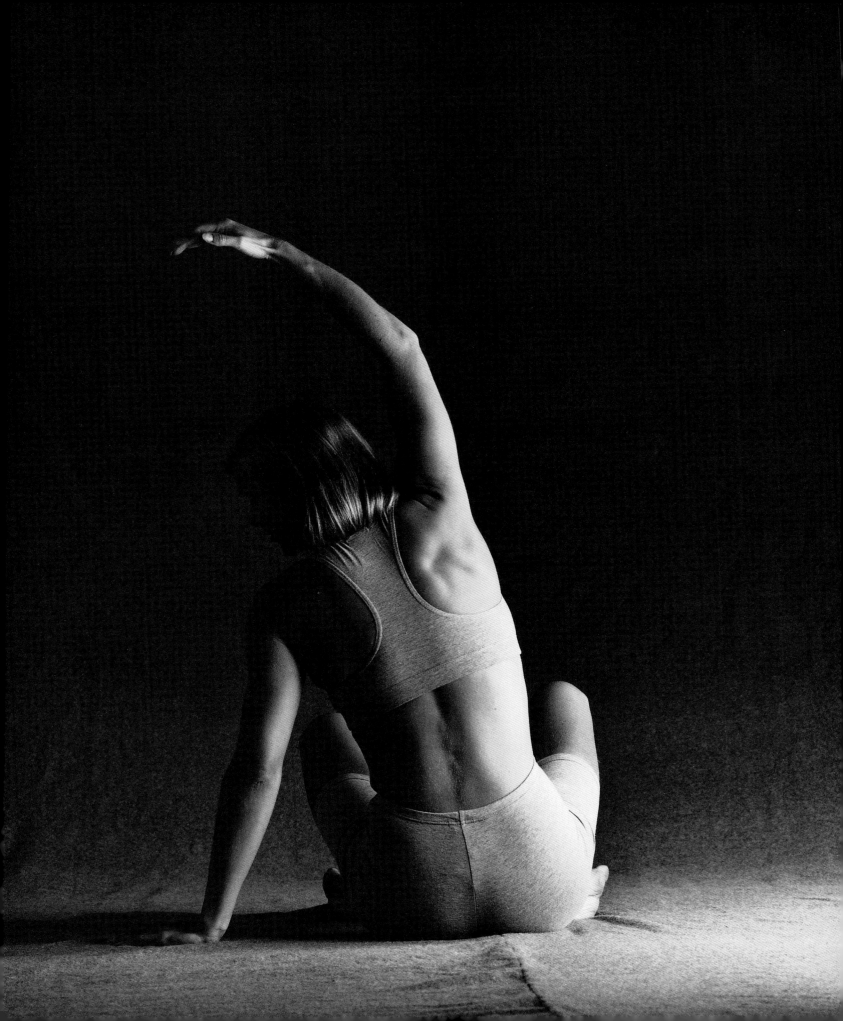

Warm-ups

Your warm-up should take five to ten minutes, although if the room is cool or if you are feeling stiff or sluggish, take a little longer to make sure your body is properly prepared.

Make your movements as big as possible to take each joint through its full range of motion. Work at a pace that allows you to control all the movements and to flow one into the other. At first, changes from one move to another might be a little rough, but don't worry about this. As you become familiar with the exercises, they will start to flow – you can even put on some music to help your mood and pace. It is probably easier, in the beginning, to learn the leg and foot movements first, adding the arms once you are comfortable.

Finally, make sure everything you need for your exercise session is close by before you start your warm-up, so you will have fewer distractions and interruptions.

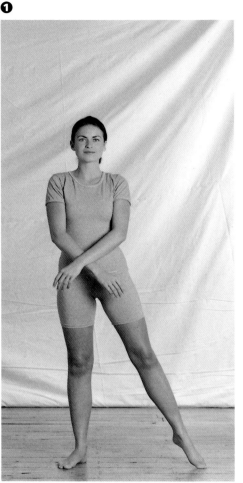

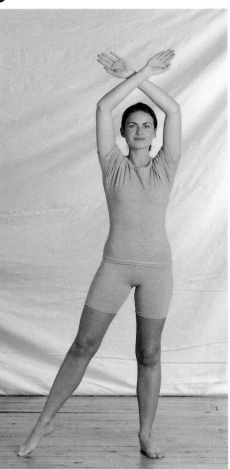

Press and heel lift

With your feet more than shoulders' width apart and slightly turned out, bend your knees, pressing both feet into the floor. Your weight should be balanced over both feet. As you straighten your legs, lift the heel of your left foot from the floor, transferring most of your weight onto your right leg and keeping your back straight. Return to the starting position by transferring your weight back over both feet, then repeat on the other side.

When you are comfortable, add the arm movements. You can roll your shoulders backward for eight counts, then change direction and roll them forward for eight counts (1). Once your shoulders have loosened up, try circling your arms in front of your body (2), then reverse the circles.

❶   ❷

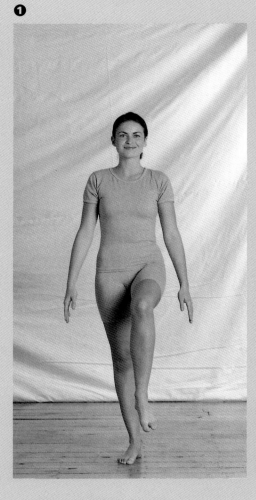 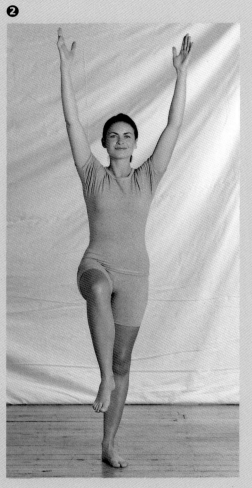

Stationary march

Maintaining good posture and alignment, gently march on the spot, staying light on your feet and letting your arms swing naturally by your side. March for 32 beats, moving back and forth if you want to. Once you establish your rhythm, you can add the arm movements. When your arms are down, exhale (1), then inhale as you raise them (2).

Pace yourself, synchronizing your feet and your breathing, taking four beats to inhale and four beats to exhale.

❶

❷

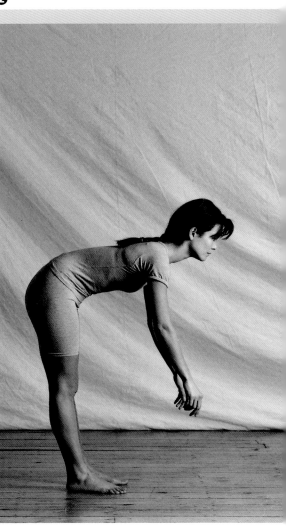

Cobra bow
Standing with feet hips' width apart, resting your fists in the small of your back, arch backward (1). Keep your head facing to the front, so you do not throw it backward. Straighten up, then curl forward from the waist, letting your arms fall freely (2). Do not push this stretch too far – your back and thighs should feel comfortable throughout. Return to standing and relax. Repeat six times.

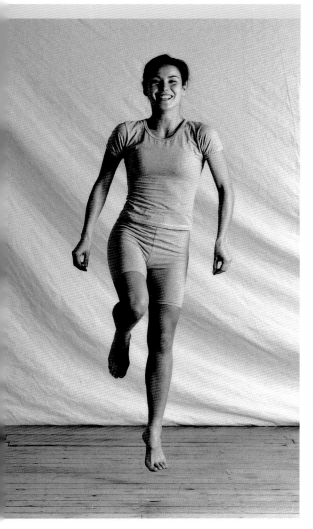

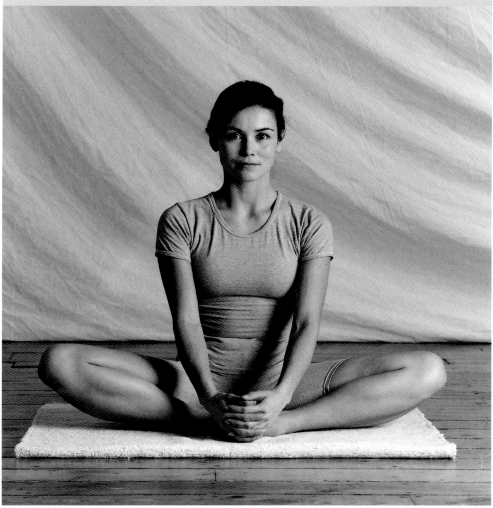

Grasshopper

This simple exercise works the lower back, buttocks, calf, and thigh muscles. Balancing on your right leg, gently hop, allowing your hip and knee to bend through a comfortable range. Hop 10 times on one leg, then 10 times on the other leg.

Butterfly

Sit on the floor, knees bent, so the soles of your feet rest against each other. Reach down with your hands and hold your ankles or your feet. Sit tall, allowing your knees to fall out. You should feel a stretch in your inner thighs and low back. Hold this position for 15 seconds, before relaxing and repeating three times.

Prayer

Kneel on the floor with your weight divided equally over your hands and knees. Shift your body back, keeping your hands flat on the floor, and curling your chin down onto your chest. Hold the stretch for 10 seconds before returning to the starting position and repeating three times.

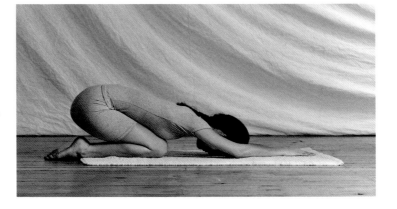

Advanced crawl

Resting on your hands and knees, keep your back stable and your weight balanced over both of your hands and left knee as you bend your right knee up toward your chest and tuck your chin down, curling your back (1). Then, extend your right leg out behind you and lift your head, making sure your back remains straight and strong (2). Repeat six times with the right leg, then six times with the left. This will improve the suppleness of your whole spine.

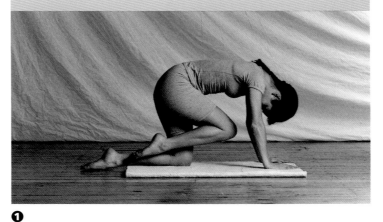

❶

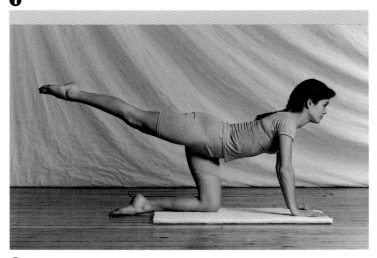

❷

Star jumps

This is a good exercise to do toward the end of your sporting warm-up. It will increase your heart rate, improve the blood flow to your arms and legs, and make the muscles in your back, buttocks, and thighs work to support your spine.

Standing with your weight equally divided over both legs, jump up in the air at the same time as you open your legs and throw both your arms up above your head. You may clap your hands above your head as you do this.

Land on the floor with feet still apart and hands above your head, then jump up into the air again, bringing your feet together and your arms back down by your sides, before landing again.

Repeat for a few minutes. You may increase the speed of the exercise as you get stronger and fitter.

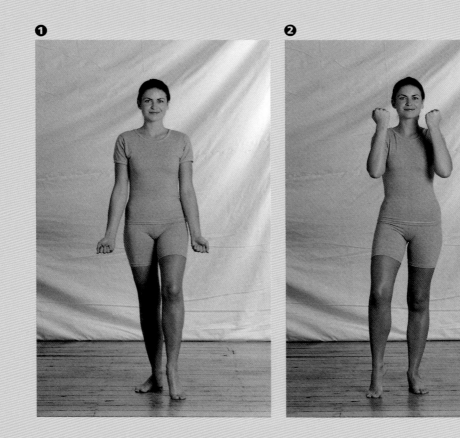

Touch and curl

Starting with your feet a little more than shoulders' width apart and slightly turned out, step your right foot in to your left foot, lightly touching the floor with your toe as your feet come together. Step out and forward with your right foot, placing your whole foot on the floor, and then step in with your left foot.

Repeat the movement from side to side, adding the arm movements. As you step to one side, straighten your arms, forming loose fists with your hands (1). As you step to the other side, bend your elbows so that your fists come up toward your shoulders, keeping your elbows fairly close to your waist (2).

Side lunge

With your feet just more than shoulders' width apart and slightly turned out, bend your knees, pressing both feet into the floor. Shift your weight to the right, bending your right knee and keeping your left leg straight. The knee of your bent leg should be over your ankle, with your knee and foot pointing in the same direction – if your knee extends over your toes, move your feet wider apart. Your hips and chest should face forward, without twisting. Return your weight to the center before shifting it to the left.

Add the arm movements: as you lunge to the right, reach for the ceiling with your left arm, and as you lunge to the left reach up with your right arm. Aim for a long line from your ankle through to the tips of your fingers. Repeat 16 times.

Lunge backs

Start with your feet hips' width apart. Push your right foot out behind you and tap the floor once with your toes, then repeat with the left leg, gradually increasing the distance between your feet as you lunge back.

Then add the arm movements. Making loose fists, bend your elbows and raise them behind you, tucking your fists under your armpits. As you lunge back, straighten your arms, pushing them behind you, then bend your elbows as your feet come together. Repeat 32 times.

❶ **❷**

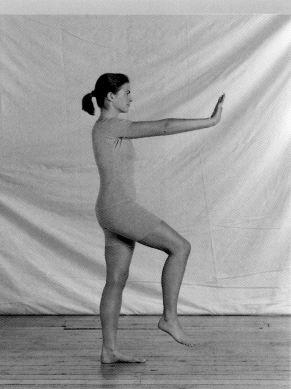

Knee lift and press

Starting with your feet a little more than shoulders' width apart and slightly turned out, shift your weight to the left, lifting your right knee slightly, keeping it lower than your hip.

Add the arm movements: bend your elbows at the side of your body, keeping them close to your chest, turning your palms out (1). When you lift your knee, extend your arms and push out with the palms of your hands (2). As you lower your knee, pull your arms back to your body. Repeat 16 times.

❶ **❷**

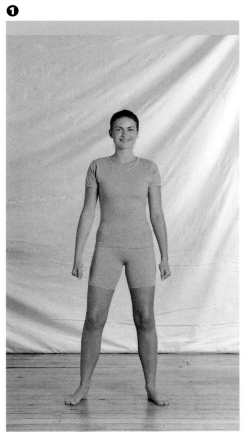

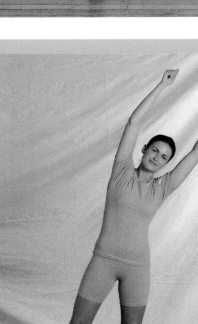

Side lift and punch

With your feet a little more than shoulders' width apart and slightly turned out, bend your knees slightly, pressing both feet into the floor. Your body weight should be balanced over both feet. As you straighten your legs, shift your weight to the left, raising your right leg out to the side, keeping your toes and hips facing forward.

Add your arms: as you bend your knees, punch toward the floor with your fists (1). As you straighten your legs, extend your arms high above your head and stretch to the side opposite your extended leg, breathing deeply (2). Repeat 16 times.

Cool-downs

A cool-down can take between 10 and 15 minutes out of every hour's exercise. As a general guideline, the more rigorous your exercise session, the longer your cool-down should be. Begin with the same type of movements you used in the warm-up, done at a much slower pace, then move on to stretches.

Finish with some conscious breathing. A few deep breaths as you stand and stretch as tall as you can will leave you feeling strong and vibrant, and a longer spell of floor relaxation, enjoying deep breathing, will make you feel peaceful and luxurious.

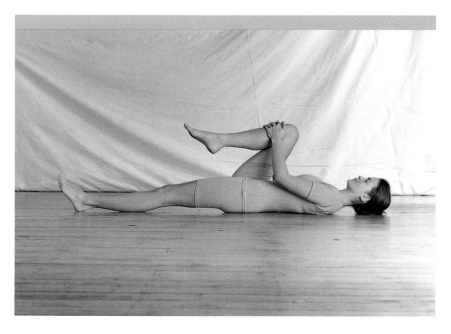

Hip flexor stretch
Lying on your back, bring your right knee to your chest, clasping it lightly. Gently press your left leg to the floor as you pull your right knee closer to your chest. Hold for 30 seconds before repeating with the other leg.

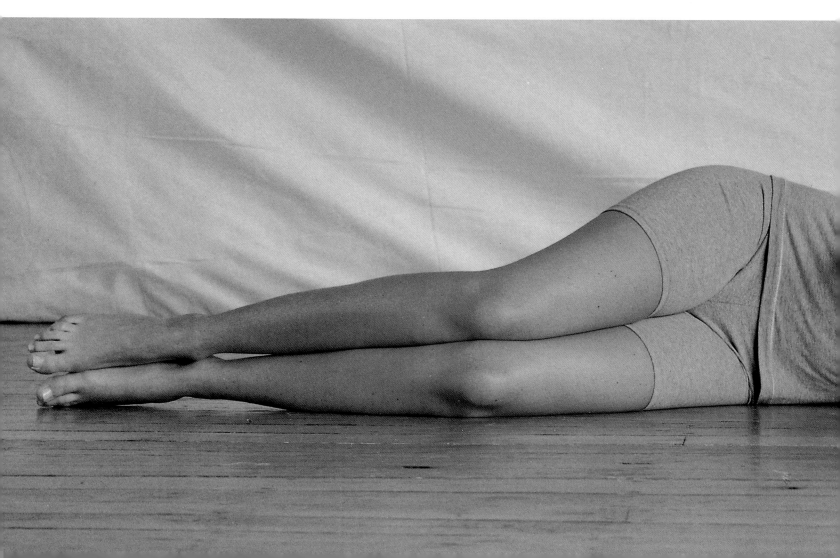

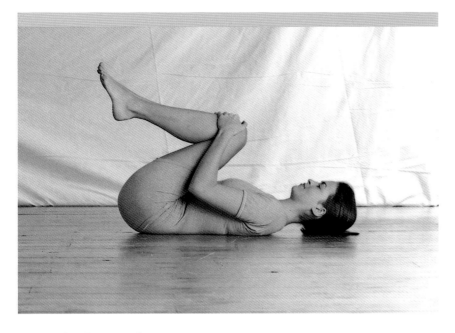

Lower back stretch

Lying on your back, keeping your neck long, hug your knees toward your chest. Your hips will rise slightly off the floor. Hold this position for around 30 seconds before lowering your legs slowly to the floor.

Floor relaxation

Lying on the floor on your side, with your knees slightly bent, and supporting your head either on your arm or with a folded towel or a pillow, close your eyes and focus on your breathing. Inhale and exhale deeply, imagining that the new air is cleansing and energizing, and that the old air takes away with it stress and fatigue. After around five minutes, start to rouse yourself gradually. If you stand up too fast, you may feel dizzy, so take your time.

Hips and Thighs

The hip and thigh muscles respond well to toning and stretching. This program provides a complete exercise system to improve the condition and appearance of these problem areas of the body. You can use the dedicated chapters to work on the hips and thighs alone, or work through the whole book for a complete toning program. To get the most from the effort you are making, bear in mind that you can boost your efforts by following a healthy diet.

You do not need a separate warm-up before beginning the Core Exercises (see page 38) or the Total Body Workout (see page 56), but remember to work gently at the start of your exercise until your muscles begin to feel free.

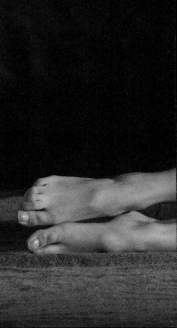

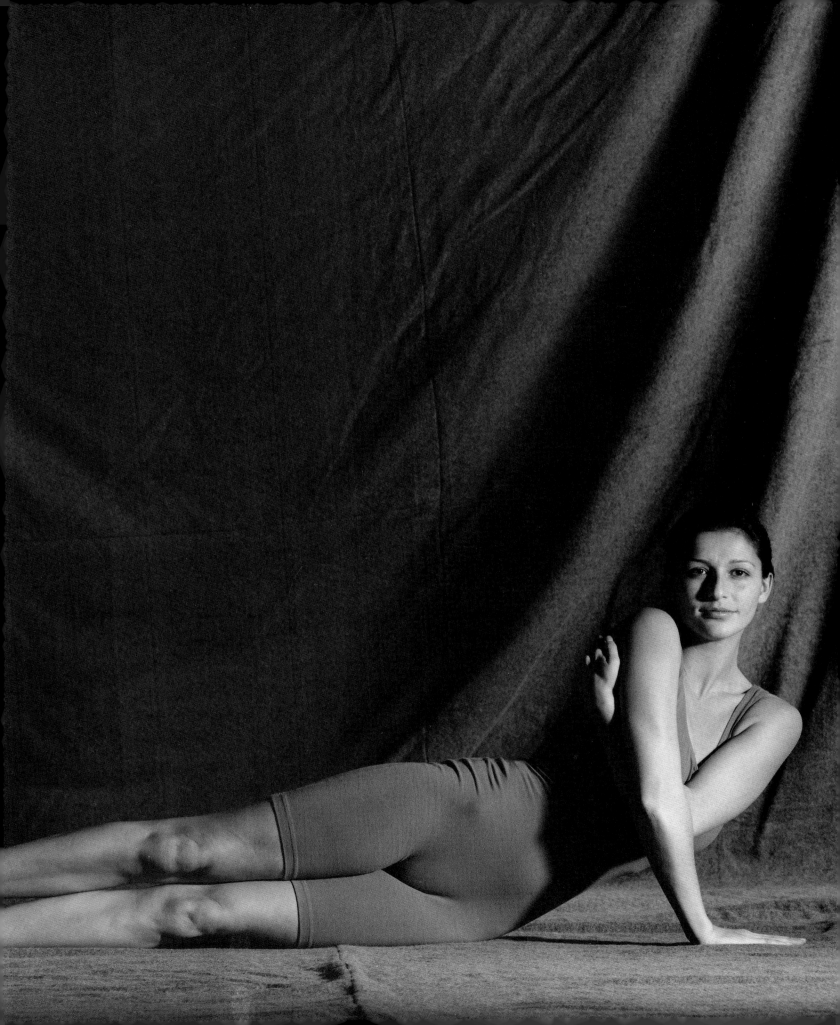

Winning the war:
the fight against cellulite

Do women have to admit defeat in the war against cellulite? No, certainly not. With the correct approach, there is a lot you can do to improve the appearance of the areas where cellulite has developed. But the many expensive magic remedies on the market today may not offer the answers. The solution can be cheaper, easier, and much closer to home.

In order to understand how to improve the appearance of your hips and thighs, it helps to understand the physiology of your body.

In both men and women, fat makes up a percentage of our body weight, and it is stored throughout the body, not just in the places you most notice its appearance. The balance of hormones in a woman's body means that she has nearly twice the volume of fat compared to an average man.

The distribution of fat on a woman's body is also different. It is to a large extent controlled by estrogen levels (estrogen is one of the most significant female sex hormones). Estrogen levels vary through our life cycle, which means that the way that our body distributes excess fat also varies. In your teens and 20s, excess weight is evenly distributed; in your 30s and 40s you tend to put it on your hips and thighs; and as you get older, you tend to put it on your waist.

The way in which the body stores fat is also determined hormonally. This is why women, unfortunately, suffer from cellulite and men in general do not.

Cellulite is not a different kind of fat – fat is fat. However, it has a different appearance in men than in women, particularly in certain notorious trouble spots, like the back of the thighs and the upper arms.

There is a marked difference in the structure of men's and women's skin, and especially in the connective tissue that runs between the layers of skin. This connective tissue builds chambers around which subcutaneous fat, the deeper layers of fat, are stored. In women the chambers created by connective tissue are more vertical than in men, so they are less adaptable to change. This means that when they become full, instead of bulging at the sides, the walls remain firm, and extra fat protrudes from the top. With age, the connective tissue becomes stronger and the

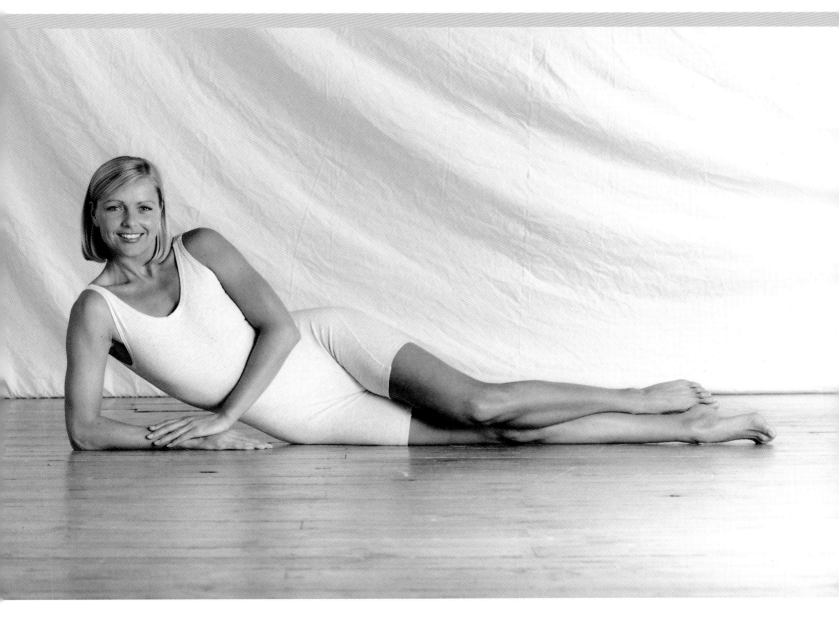

As you improve the muscle tone of your hips and thighs, you will find that they begin to appear firmer and more shapely.

skin becomes thinner, exaggerating the effect of cellulite. In men the connective tissue builds a structure akin to a honeycomb, which is a more flexible arrangement.

Many of the costly cellulite remedies marketed today, such as creams and massage mitts, will certainly help you to improve the condition of your skin. This is beneficial, as if your skin is firmer and smoother, the appearance of cellulite will lessen somewhat. However, these techniques have not been shown to have any effect on the underlying causes of the appearance of cellulite – they cannot change the structure of connective tissue, which is genetically determined, nor can they eliminate the fat stored in the body.

The only long-term solution to this age-old problem is exercise combined with a healthy diet. This will help tone and firm your hips and thighs. You will reduce the percentage of fat stored in your body by burning more energy than you take in with your diet.

Controlling the process

The combination of exercise and diet can also affect the way your body processes and stores fat in a more fundamental sense.

The way the body handles fat is determined by the levels of a number of hormones and enzymes. While much of this is out of our control, being part of the body's process of homeostasis, or internal self-regulation, we can take steps to control the ease with which the body stores, rather than uses, fat.

Diet is one line of defense. Cutting back on the amount of fat in your diet has two positive effects. One is, obviously, that if your body is supplied with less fat, it has less fat to store. It is also less likely to store the fat with which it is supplied, using it for essential metabolic processes instead.

Exercise is also your ally. You not only burn calories, helping you to balance your food intake with your body's needs, but you also reduce the activity of the enzymes that cause your body to store fat.

Be aware, however, that it is dangerous to cut too much fat from your diet. The human body needs a certain amount of fat and responds badly to being deprived: if you go on a "starvation" diet, totally cutting out fat (and therefore drastically limiting calories as well), your body will do all it can to conserve energy,

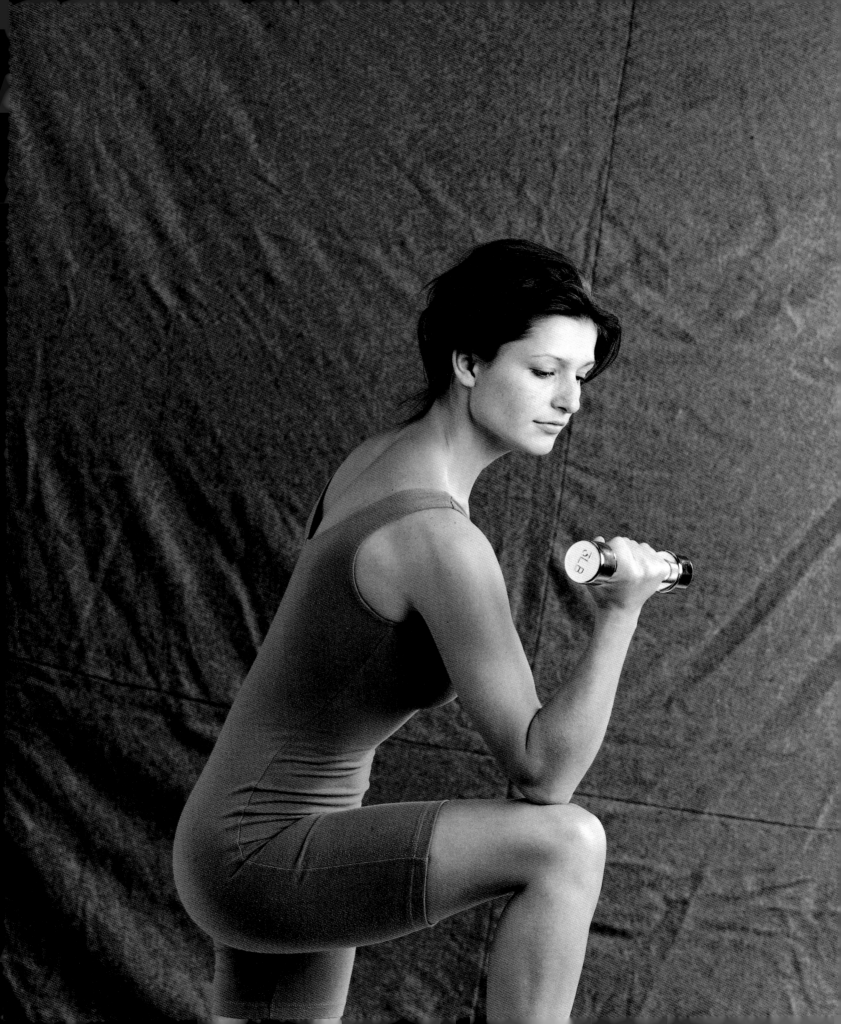

protecting its fat stores. This will make it harder to lose weight. In addition, excessive thinness carries its own dangers: it is linked to early death in both men and women, and to menstrual irregularity in women, which increases the risk of osteoporosis, or gradual weakening of the bones.

However, excess fat is also linked to a number of diseases, including heart disease and various forms of cancer in both men and women. If you are overweight, even a small weight loss, of only five or ten per cent of body weight can be enough to lessen the risk of these health problems.

If you ever feel dispirited, remember this little bit of good news. Some fat on the hips and thighs is actually good for you. Where you carry any excess weight also has ramifications for health. Studies have shown that a concentration of fat in the abdominal area is a greater health risk than a concentration of fat around the hips and thighs. This extra fat on the abdomen has been linked to certain types of cancer (including breast cancer and endometrial cancer), high blood pressure, heart disease and even diabetes. So beware of yo-yo dieting – the cycle of losing weight by

following strict diets, then putting the weight back on soon after. It can alter your natural distribution, causing you to gain weight on your abdomen.

Nor should you be seduced by the various detoxifying diet plans suggested specifically to tackle the problem of cellulite. Keep in mind that cellulite is a natural development in a woman's body – it does not result from an unnatural build-up of toxins. While a short, sensible detoxifying program may be revitalizing, it is not a long-term solution.

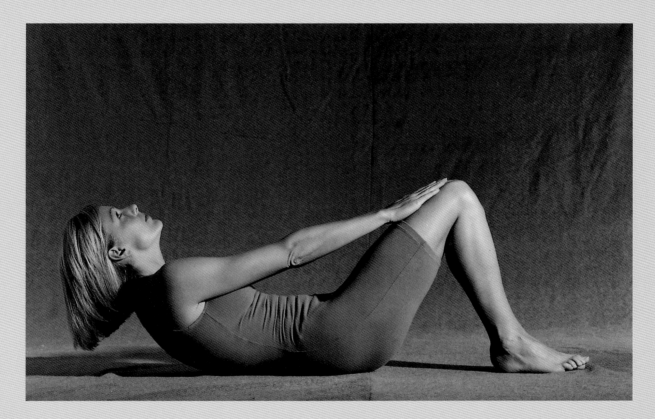

The right kind of targeted exercise, in combination with a healthy diet, will help you to improve the appearance of your hips and thighs, toning and firming these trouble spots.

Body facts

The muscles in the hips, thighs, and buttocks are some of the largest in the body, and also some of the hardest-working. They are integral in many of our regular activities, including walking, sitting, standing, and climbing stairs, so their condition is of prime importance to our overall fitness and health.

In order to tone these muscles effectively by stretching and strengthening them, it is important to understand where they are, how they are inter-related, and how they work.

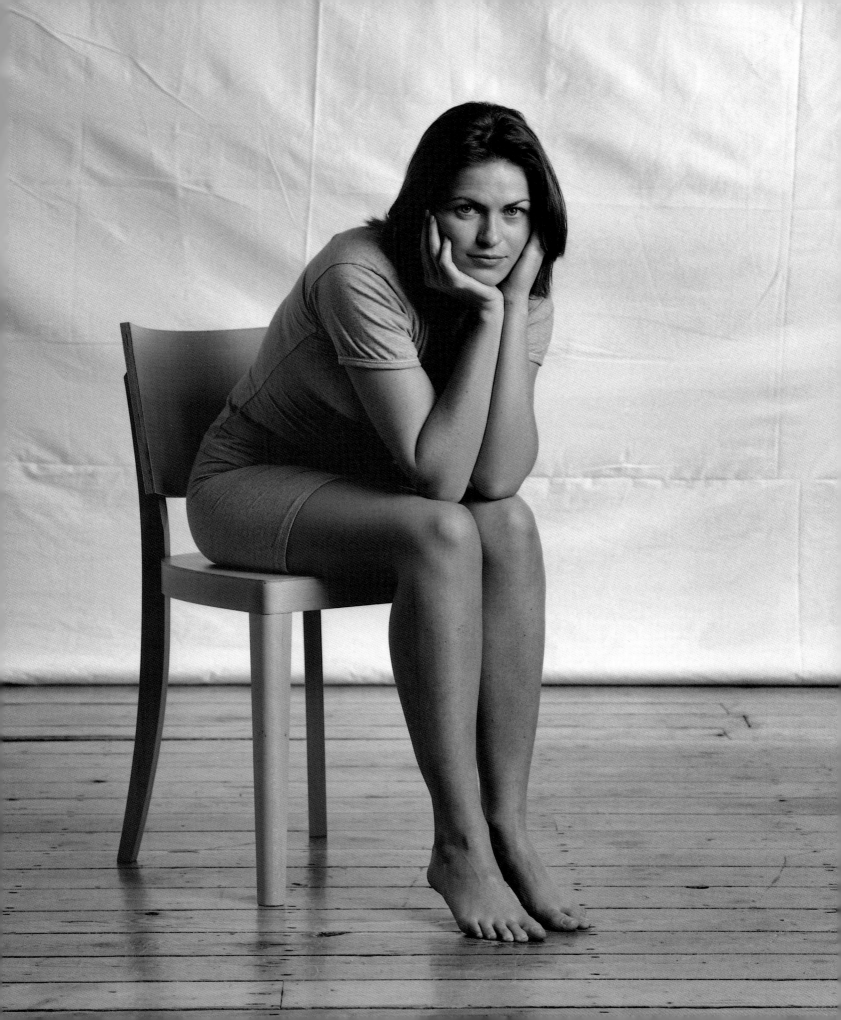

Body facts: hips, thighs, and buttocks

Our hips, thighs, and buttocks contain some of the body's strongest muscles and also some of the most vigorously used. They are involved in many activities, including walking, climbing stairs, and sitting down and standing up. They are also integral in establishing the stability of the torso.

The intricate arrangement of the bones of the lower body means that we require very little actual muscle activity to stand upright – we are designed to balance.

The pelvic girdle – the correct name for the hipbones – connects the torso and legs, supports the internal organs, and balances the trunk. It consists actually of three bones, which fuse in early adulthood. A woman's pelvis is wider than a man's, to allow for the birth canal.

The muscles at the front of the thigh are known as the quadriceps and, as the name suggests, there are four parts to the group. At the top, three are directly attached to the femur, or thigh bone, and one is attached to the pelvis. At the lower end, the muscles form the patella tendon, which is attached to the kneecap. These muscles work to straighten your knees, and as part of that function, they also protect your knees by maintaining the position of your kneecaps.

Working in opposition to the quadriceps are the hamstrings, a group of three muscles in back of each thigh. This muscle group assists in straightening the body at the hip joint and in bending the knee. In most people, the hamstrings are smaller and weaker than the quadriceps. This imbalance means that they are more prone to injury. In addition, tightness in the hamstrings reduces the mobility of the hip joint, increasing strain on the lower back.

While all the muscles in our legs suffer from a sedentary lifestyle, the hamstring muscles suffer most from the inactivity. They shorten, making them tight, less efficient, and more prone to injury. It is essential to stretch this muscle group carefully during your warm-up not only when you run or play any sports, but also when you exercise at home.

It also is a good idea occasionally to focus specifically on your hamstring muscles (see pages 52–53) during workouts when you are working on your hips and thighs.

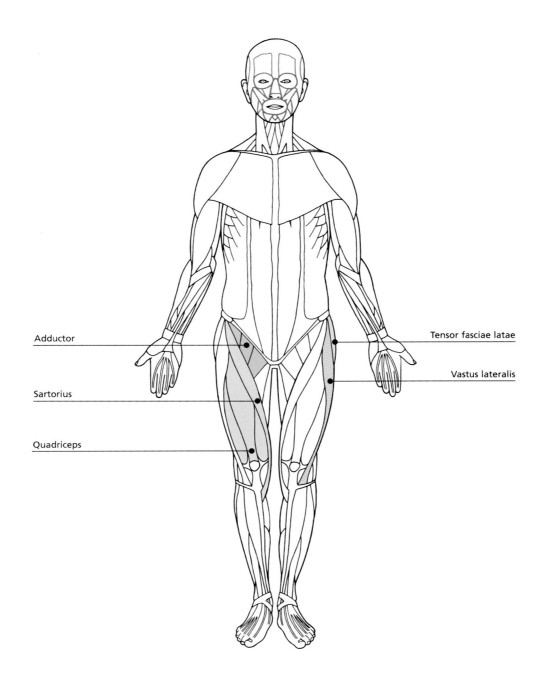

Adductor

Tensor fasciae latae

Sartorius

Vastus lateralis

Quadriceps

Front of the body

The quadriceps are the major muscles at the front of the thigh. They are a group of four muscles: three are attached directly to the thighbone and one is attached to the pelvic girdle (the hipbones). All four attach to the patella tendon, which connects to the kneecaps. The other muscles at the front of the thigh work to move your legs laterally, or sideways: the adductors move the leg toward the midline of the body and the abductors, the muscles on the outside of the thigh, move the leg *away*.

Just as the muscles of the front and back of the thigh work in opposition, so do the muscles of the inner and outer thigh. The outer thigh muscles are known as the abductors. These lift or move your legs laterally away from the midline of your body. The inner thigh muscles are known as the adductors, and they work to bring your legs together and to move them across the midline of the body when necessary. They attach the front of the pelvis to the femur, stabilizing the torso when you walk.

The hip flexors are the muscles that work specifically when you bend at the hip – for example, when you sit down or when you climb a step. Tight hip flexors can cause your back to arch excessively as the upper body is pulled forward constantly.

The main muscle of the buttocks, the gluteus maximus, is the largest in the body, and it forms the shape of the buttocks. Working in opposition to the hip flexors, this muscle is active when you straighten up at the hip joint – for example, when you climb stairs or when you stand up from sitting.

The hip joint is a ball-and-socket joint, like the shoulder. This means that it is designed for rotational motion, although its range of motion is more restricted than that of the shoulder. It is more flexible in bending forward than it is in bending backward, helping to ensure our stability when we are standing. This rotational motion is necessary for walking: when your right foot touches the ground in walking, the right hip joint rotates externally at the same time as the left hip joint rotates internally. The hip rotators, along with the gluteus muscles, are designed to control this rotational movement.

One of the reasons it is important to keep the muscles of the hips and thighs in good condition is that the hip joint bears a lot of force when you are walking or running. The muscles have to support the joint adequately, allowing it to bear the force more easily by taking advantage of its full range of motion.

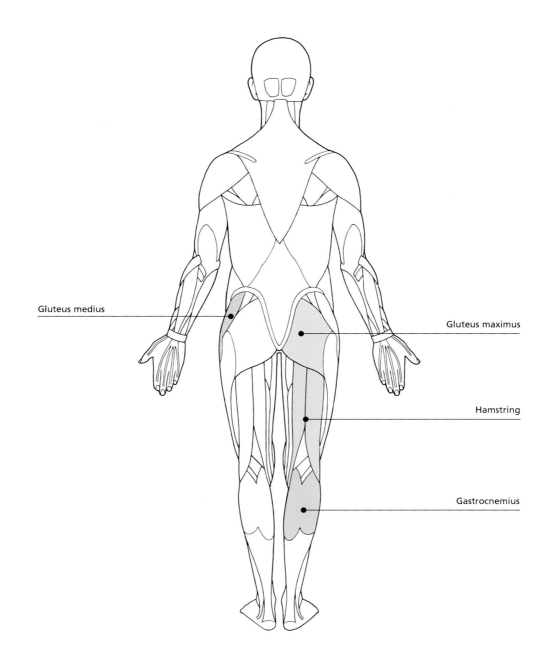

Gluteus medius

Gluteus maximus

Hamstring

Gastrocnemius

Back of the body

The gluteus maximus is the largest muscle in the body and forms the shape of the buttocks. Appearance is not the only reason to keep this muscle in shape: it is also involved in many activities, including climbing stairs and standing up from a sitting position.

The hamstring muscles are the major muscles of the rear thigh. In many people, they are shortened owing to inactivity and wearing high-heeled or restrictive shoes, and can therefore be uncomfortable. The same may be true of the gastrocnemius, the calf muscle.

Core exercises

These core exercises have been designed to work all the major muscle groups of the hips and thighs in a balanced manner, focusing on both stretch and strength. This way, your muscles can become firmer and tighter without growing bulky – stretching will help your muscles retain their length and take on a more desirable shape.

Balance your exercises between opposing body parts. For example, if you choose a strength exercise for the outer thigh, you should choose one for the inner thigh. You should also complement each strength exercise with a stretch to relax the muscles.

Don't expect immediate results – it takes the body six to eight weeks to adapt. Try to do this type of workout at least twice a week, aiming for a total time of 60 to 75 minutes. However, if 20 to 30 minutes is all you can spare, go for it anyway.

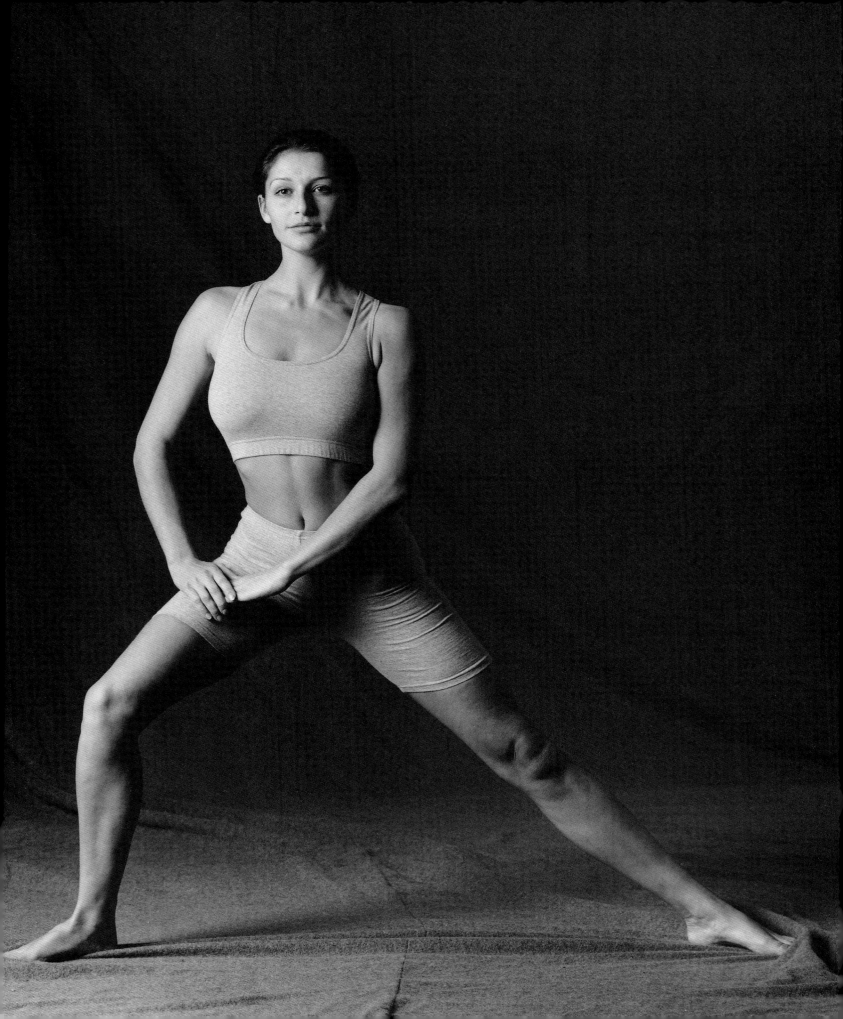

Outer thigh

The outer thigh muscles, or abductors, move your leg sideways away from the midline of your body, so to strengthen those muscles, you must move the leg in that direction, lifting the working leg to a 45° angle. Start at a slow pace, perhaps four beats to lift and four beats to lower, but you can vary this rhythm – it is more challenging to work slowly.

You can do this kind of exercise from a variety of positions: standing, kneeling, or lying. The kneeling position is the most advanced because it requires a lot of abdominal and back strength. If you try this and feel any strain, especially in your lower back, try one of the other options.

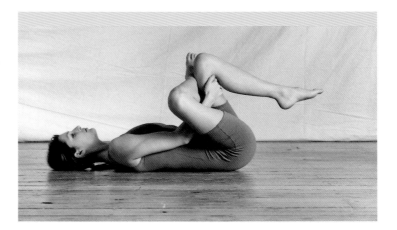

Heel-on-thigh stretch
Lie on your back with your left knee bent and your left foot on the floor. Rest the heel of your right foot on the thigh of your left leg so your right knee is pointing out to the right side. Keeping your left knee bent and your head and shoulders relaxed and on the floor, place both hands around your left thigh and pull it up and in toward your chest. You should feel a stretch along the right outer thigh. Hold this for at least 20 seconds.

❶

❷

Cross-legged stretch
Standing tall, cross your left foot closely behind your right foot, keeping both feet flat on the floor and the outside edges of your feet touching (1). Bend your right knee and, keeping your left leg straight, push your left hip out to the left side until you feel a stretch in your left buttock and along your left thigh (2). Although pushing out your hip will cause your torso to lean slightly in the opposite direction, try to keep your torso as long and strong as you can.

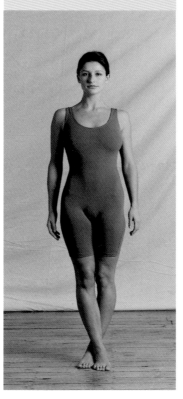

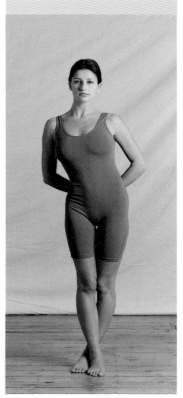

❶

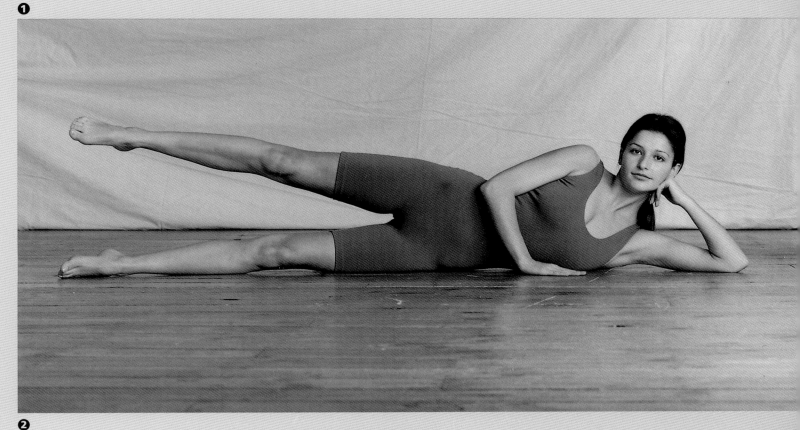

❷

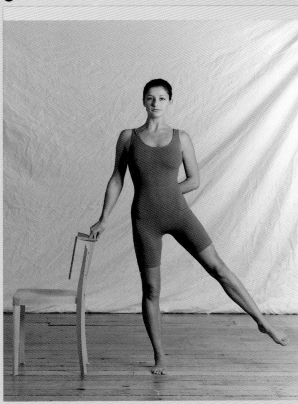

Side leg lift

Lie on your left side, keeping your body as long and extended as possible and making sure that your right hip is directly above your left hip. Place your right hand on the floor close to your chest to stabilize yourself. With a controlled movement, lift and lower your right leg as many times as you can, working toward at least 20 repetitions (1). To enhance the effectiveness of this exercise, lower your right leg to just above your left leg and immediately start the next lift, keeping a little tension in the muscles of your right leg through the movement.

You can also do this exercise while standing, using a chair or the wall as support (2). Remember to make sure that your hips are facing forward and your body is upright.

As an advanced variation, you can use ankle weights for added resistance.

Inner thigh

Your inner thigh muscles, known as adductors, work to bring your legs together and, if necessary, to move them past the midline of your body. These muscles may be stronger than the abductors of your outer thigh, because they are used more often. In order to tone the adductors, you have to repeat their usual movement but working against the downward force of gravity. This principle also applies to exercises that tone and strengthen the outer thighs.

To keep yourself motivated, you can vary the positions, doing these exercises standing, lying, or kneeling – standing is the easiest option, and kneeling is the most difficult. Aim to do at least 20 repetitions without resting.

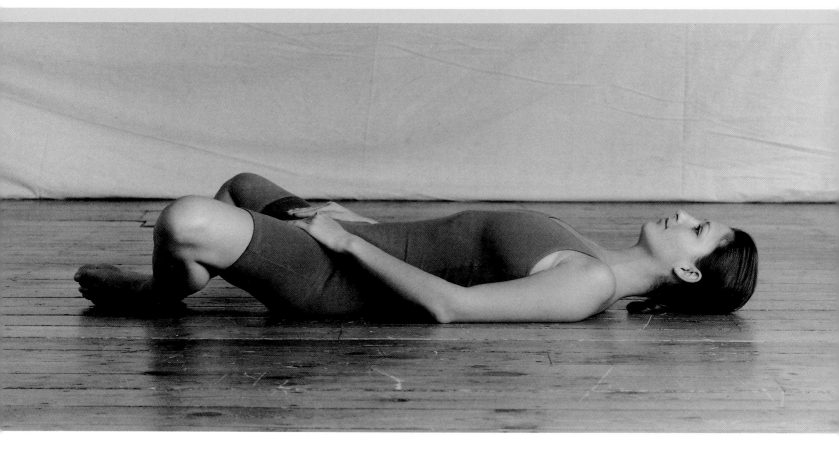

Diamond
Lie on your back with your knees bent and the soles of your feet touching. Have your heels as close to your buttocks as is comfortable, and aim to bring your knees as close as you can to the floor. Your lower back does not have to be pressed into the floor, so allow it to curve naturally. You should feel a stretch along your inner thighs. To increase the stretch, use your hands to push down gently on your thighs. Hold the stretch for at least 20 seconds. You can also do this stretch while sitting.

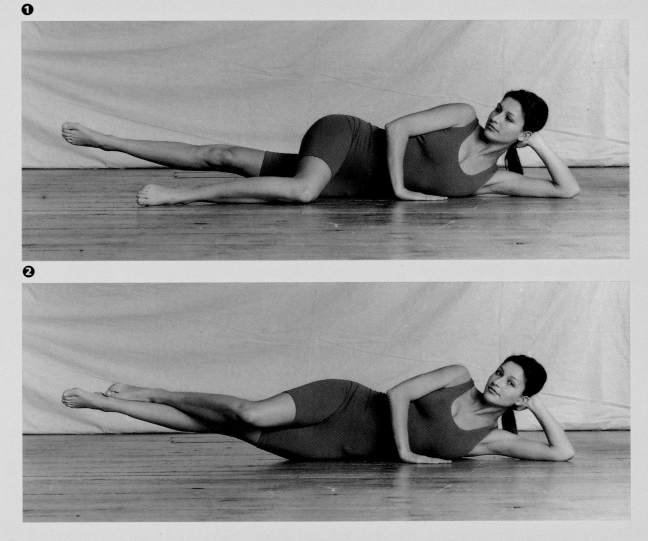

Lying lower leg lift

Lie on the floor on your left side with your legs stretched out, placing your right hand in front of your body to stabilize your torso, and rest your head on your left arm. Bend your right knee to a 90° angle and place it on the floor in front of you, so that your knee is in line with your hips. Lift your left leg, keeping it straight (1), and lower it until it nearly touches the floor before lifting it again. By keeping it slightly off the floor, you are maintaining tension in your leg, making the exercise more challenging. Breathe in as you lift your leg and out as you lower it, keeping the movements smooth and regular. Aim to repeat this around 20 times before resting and then switching sides.

For an advanced variation, rest your right leg on your left leg (2) so that as you lift your leg, you are working against the force of gravity with more of your body's weight.

❶

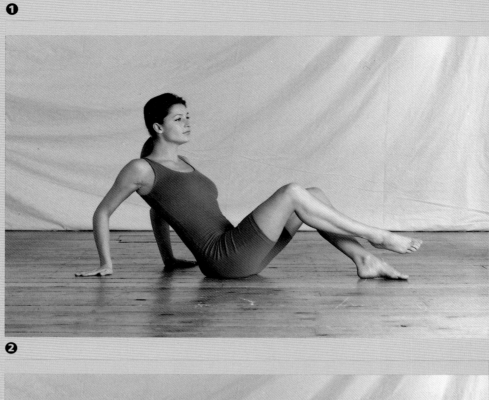

❷

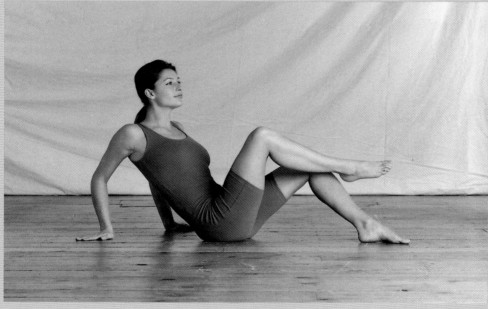

Seated leg hook

Sit on the floor, leaning back slightly with your knees bent, and place your hands behind you to stabilize your torso. Bring the heel of your right foot in front of the ankle of your left leg, and turn your right leg out so your inner thigh is almost facing the ceiling (1). Keeping a distance of an inch (2.5cm) between heel and shin, lift and lower your right heel up and down the length of your left shin (2).

Standing leg cross

This is a very gentle exercise for your inner thighs. Standing with your left foot slightly in front of your right leg with a chair or a wall for support, lift your left leg as far as possible across the midline of your body, and then lower your leg to the starting position. Make sure your hips are parallel and facing forward throughout. Repeat this as many times as you can, building up to at least 20 times, before changing legs. If you have ankle weights, wear them to increase the challenge.

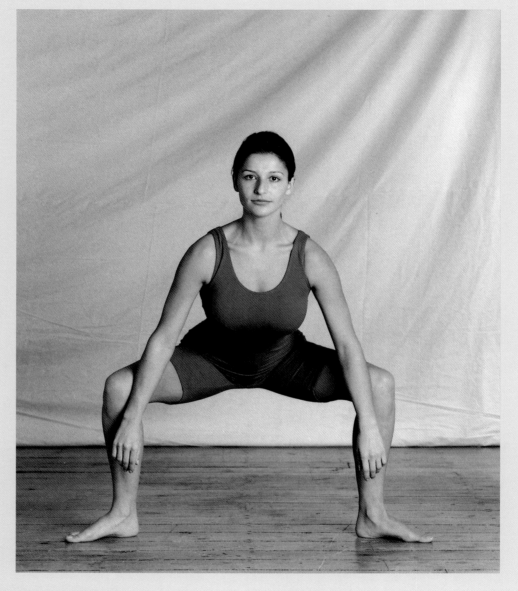

Plié press back

Standing with your feet a little more than shoulders' distance apart, turn your feet out, keeping your knees directly over your ankles and your knees and feet pointing in the same direction. Bend your knees, sticking your bottom out behind you, as you lower your hips almost to the level of your knees. Placing your forearms on the inside of your thighs, push gently against your thighs to increase the stretch. Make sure that your back is straight, your chest is lifted, and your abdominal muscles are pulled in. Hold this stretch for around 20 seconds, then straighten up and relax.

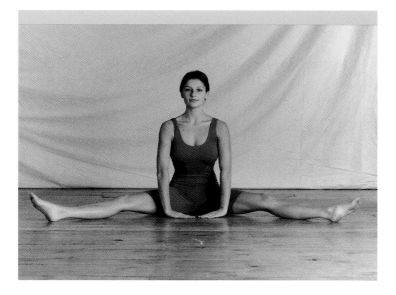

Wide V Stretch

Sitting on the floor with your legs straight out in front of you, move your legs apart until you feel an inner thigh stretch. Support yourself by placing your hands on the floor in front of you. Maintaining a long, strong back and good posture, lean forward slightly from the hips if you want to increase the stretch.

If you find this difficult, you can use gravity to help. Lie on your back and bend your knees in toward your chest, then straighten your legs up toward the ceiling. Ease your legs apart until you feel a stretch. To increase the stretch, you can press down gently with your hands on your inner thighs.

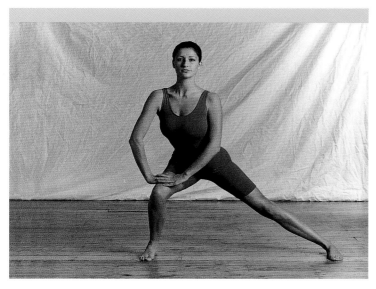

Side lunge

With your feet placed a little more than shoulders' width apart and slightly turned out, bend your right knee and shift your weight over to your right side. Try to keep your hips and chest facing forward, and check that your right knee is positioned over your ankle, your right knee and foot are facing in the same direction, and your left foot is flat on the floor. You can place your hands on the thigh of your bent leg for support, which will help you maintain the alignment of your upper body while you hold this stretch.

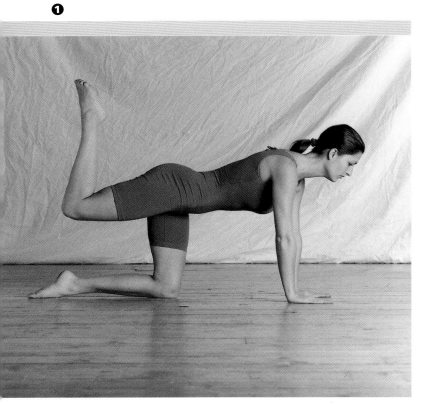

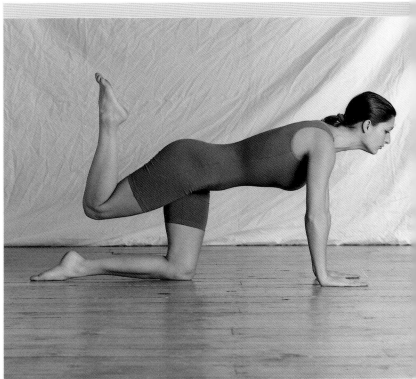

Kneeling knee cross-back

Kneel on all fours with your knees hips' distance apart. Place your forearms on the floor so your elbows are directly under your shoulders – when you are stronger, keep your arms straight. Raise your right leg straight out behind you, in line with your hip, and keeping your knee in line with your hip, bend it so your heel is toward the ceiling (1). Move your right knee across your left leg and down toward the floor (2), then lift your knee back in line with your hip. Repeat this 20 times before switching sides.

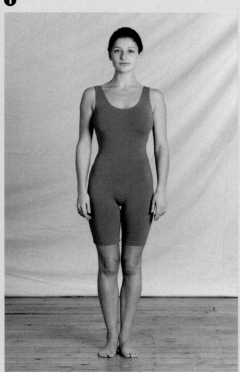 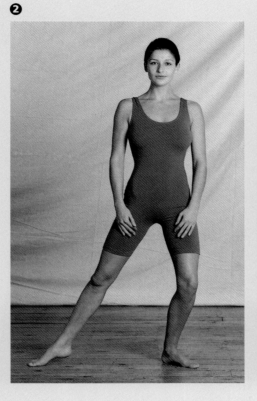 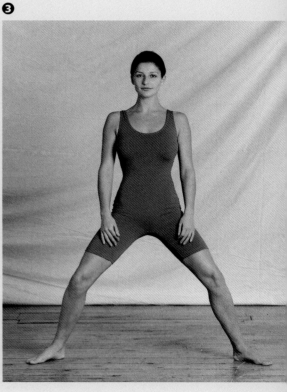

Slide

Stand with your feet together facing front (1), and step your right foot out to your right side so that your feet are at least shoulders' distance apart (2). Keeping your whole foot in contact with the floor and actually pushing your foot down on the floor, drag your right foot in toward your left foot (3) until your feet are together again. Make sure that your hips remain parallel and facing forward. Step out with your left foot and repeat on that side. Together these movements make one set.

The resistance you create by dragging your foot along the floor will make your inner thigh muscles work harder, but if you are doing this on carpet, beware of too much friction. Repeat as many times as you can, aiming for at least 20 sets.

Front thigh

The quadriceps, the muscle group located at the front of your thighs, work to straighten your knees, and they also help to protect your knees and the position of your knee caps. You must balance any strength work done on the quadriceps by also working on the hamstrings, the muscles at the back of your thighs (see pages 52–3).

You have to do most exercises for this muscle group in a standing position, unless you are working on specialized machines in a gym.

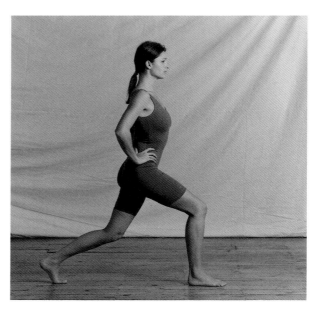

Forward lunge
Step forward two foot lengths with your right foot, and, at the same time, bend your left knee. Make sure that when you step forward, the knee of your front leg is over your ankle. If this is uncomfortable, you can shorten the distance you step forward.

❶

❷

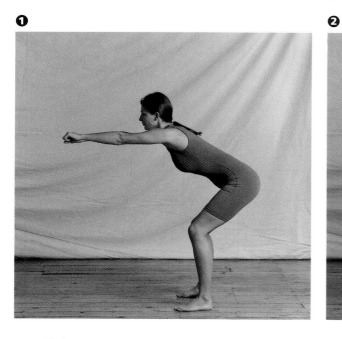

Parallel squat
Standing with your feet hips' width apart and your hands midway down your thighs for upper body support, bend your knees and slowly lower your hips down and back (but no lower than your knees) as you raise your arms until you look like a jockey on an imaginary horse. Your knees should remain above your ankles. Raise yourself upright just as slowly to a standing position. As you grow stronger, you can aim for the 20 repetition mark. To help balance, you can widen your stance slightly or hold on to a chair (2).

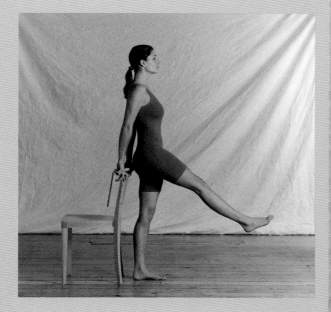

Standing leg raise

Using a chair or the wall for support, stand with your feet facing forward, a natural distance apart. Raise one leg in front of you, taking four beats to lift and the same to lower that leg. The slower the movement, the harder the muscles have to work. Repeat the action 20 times before changing legs.

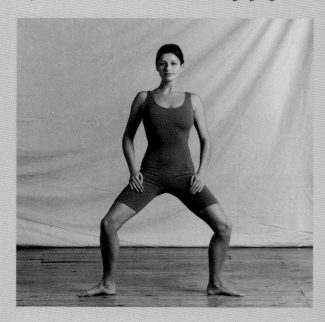

Plié squat

This is a variation of the parallel squat (opposite), with your hips open and your knees and feet turned out. Your knees should be in line with your ankles. This time, press your hips straight down and don't allow your bottom to stick out.

Quad stretch

Standing with your feet a natural distance apart, bend your right knee and lift your foot so you can clasp your ankle behind you. Tilt your bottom under slightly and try to keep your thighs close together as you pull your heel up toward your buttocks, keeping your torso strong and upright. You should feel a stretch down the front of your thigh. If you need to, use a chair or the wall for support. As a variation you can do the same stretch while lying on your stomach.

Rear thigh and buttocks

For most people, the hamstrings, at the rear of the thighs, are smaller and weaker than the quadriceps that oppose them, which makes them more susceptible to injury. You can address this imbalance with exercise. While most of the time you should do an equal number of exercises for the hamstrings and for the quadriceps, you can vary this occasionally by focusing more on the hamstrings – try doing a double set of hamstring curls after every set of front thigh exercises.

The muscles that make up your buttocks are known as the gluteus muscles, or gluts for short. With exercise, you can maintain and improve the firmness and shapeliness of your bottom. Other exercises to work these muscles are the parallel squat, the plié squat, and the forward lunge (see pages 50–51).

Seated crossover
Sit on the floor with your left leg on the floor and bent at the knee. Bend your right leg and cross it over your left leg, placing your right foot on the floor to your left. Keep your torso stabilized and your back tall as you place your left hand on the outside of your right knee and ease your knee over a little farther. Try to keep both buttocks on the floor. You will probably also feel this stretch along your outer thigh, and, if you gently twist and hold your body to look over your right shoulder, you should also feel a stretch in your lower back.

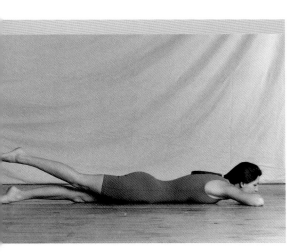

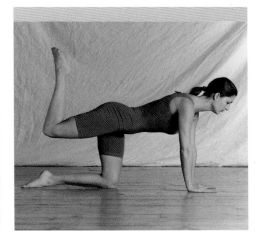

Rear leg lift

Lying face down on the floor (with your forehead resting on the back of your hands for comfort if you want), lift and lower your right leg as you keep both hipbones in contact with the floor. Focus on lifting from the top of your thigh while gently pressing your hips into the floor. If you are doing the exercise correctly, you will only be able to raise your leg a few inches off the floor. Each movement should be done in two to four beats. To make it easier, you can bend the knee of your lifting leg. Repeat the movement as many times as you can, aiming for 20 repetitions on each leg.

As an advanced variation, you can lift both legs at the same time, but great movement control is essential to protect your lower back.

Lying hamstring stretch

Lying on your back with your knees bent and your feet on the floor, pull your right thigh in toward your chest and aim to straighten your leg. Hold your thigh or your calf to support your leg.

To increase the stretch, pull gently on your leg to ease it closer to your chest. Remember, the stretch should be held for at least 20 seconds.

Hamstring curl

On all fours with your knees about hips' width apart – you should rest your forearms on the floor at first to stabilize your torso – raise your right leg straight out behind you so that your knee is aligned with your hip. Bend your knee to move your heel toward your buttocks, then straighten your leg out again. The timing of the movement should be moderate to slow, taking two to four beats to bring your heel in and the same to straighten your leg. Keep your torso stabilized and your head and neck aligned with your spine. When you have the strength in the torso to maintain good posture and your back does not sag, you can do the same exercise with straight arms, making sure you do not lock your elbows.

Hip flexors and hip rotators

Your hip flexors are generally strong because they are used whenever you bend your knees to step up, and when you bend at the hip – to sit down, for example. Tight hip flexors can cause your bottom to protrude slightly, and your back may arch as the upper body is pulled forward, causing discomfort. You can address any imbalances between strength and flexibility by doing the stretch without the strength exercise once in a while.

Your hip rotators will usually be exercised while you work other muscle groups, and they do not normally need specific attention. However, you might want to focus on them occasionally.

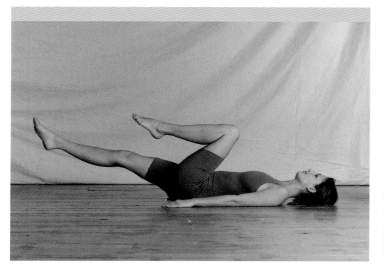

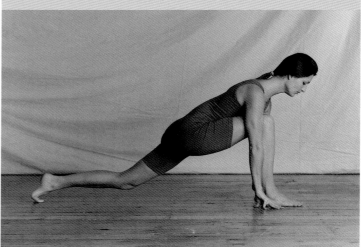

Leg extensions

Lying on the floor, bend your legs so that your knees are directly above your hips. Keeping your whole back on the floor, especially your lower back, straighten your right leg, then pull your right leg in as you extend your left leg. The motion is not cycling or circular, but a straight pressing out of your heel and a pulling in of your knee, done slowly and evenly, as if you were standing and alternately lifting your knees. Repeat the movement as many times as possible, aiming for at least 20 repetitions.

Low lunge

From a kneeling position, step your right foot forward, keeping your knee above your ankle and supporting yourself by placing your hands on the floor at either side of your right foot. Straighten your left leg behind you, keeping your toes on the floor, so you feel a stretch at the front of your hip and down the front of your thigh. Make sure you keep a straight line from your ear down to your hip. If you want to increase the stretch, you can bend your left knee slightly.

❶

❷

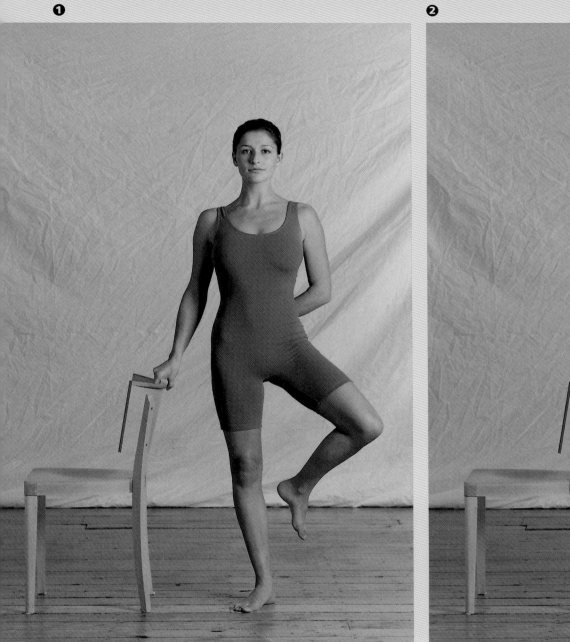

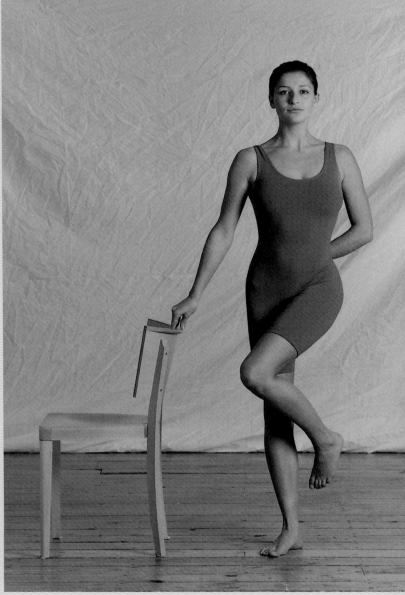

Standing hip rotation

Using a chair or a wall for support, balance on your right leg and bend your left leg at the knee and the hip. Lift your left knee up and across toward the right, then turn your leg out from the hip, moving your knee away from your body (1), then lift your left knee up and across to the right (2), in one flowing movement. Repeat at least 20 times, keeping the movement slow and even.

Total body workout

When you are targeting hips and thighs in your exercise routines, it is important not to neglect the other parts of your body. Otherwise, you could cause muscular imbalances that increase the risk of injury. It is worth paying special attention to the upper body, because women, in particular, are often comparatively weak in that area. Try to vary your exercise pattern, alternating one session where you focus exclusively on your hips and thighs with another where you can take a more holistic approach.

Although sometimes more than one exercise is presented here for a particular part of the body, choose only one or two exercises and put as much effort into those as possible. Begin by doing as many repetitions as you can, aiming, as you get stronger, for 20 without resting, and trying to hold all stretches for around 20 to 30 seconds.

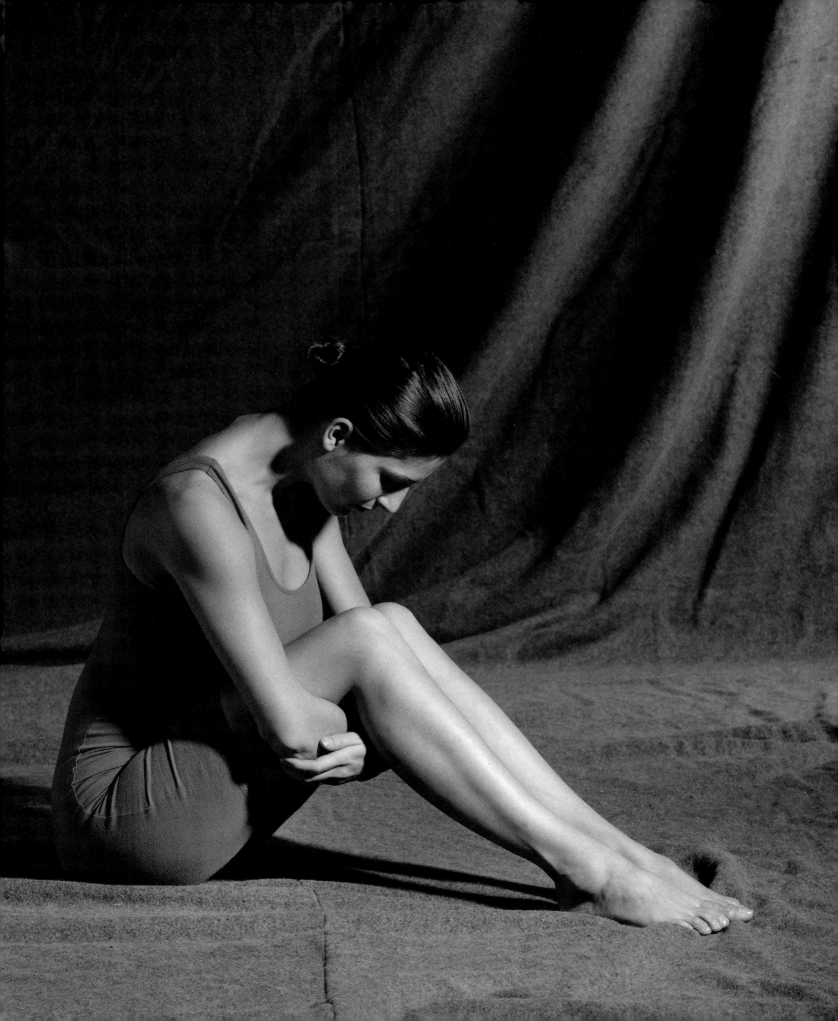

Shoulders and upper body

The muscles of your shoulders, the deltoids, are small, particularly compared to your buttocks and thighs, so they may tire easily when you first start exercising and later if you start to use weights.

Don't worry about this – rest between repetitions and ease your shoulders out with shoulder rolls and other gentle stretches. If you are suffering from stress, these stretches can also help you to relax.

❶ **❷**

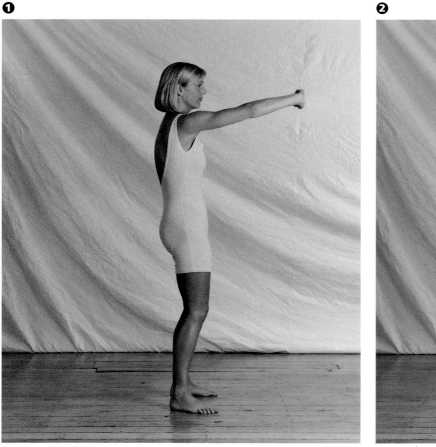

Upper body stretch

Bring your arms in front of you and link your fingers. Turn your palms out to face front and push away with your hands as you straighten your arms (1). Your back should be rounded and your shoulders rolled in as you stretch the back of your body. Then clasp your hands behind your back and raise your arms up and away from your body to stretch your front (2).

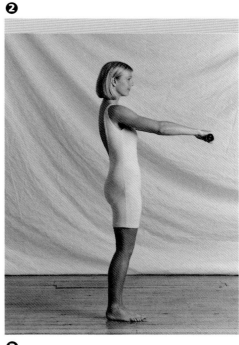

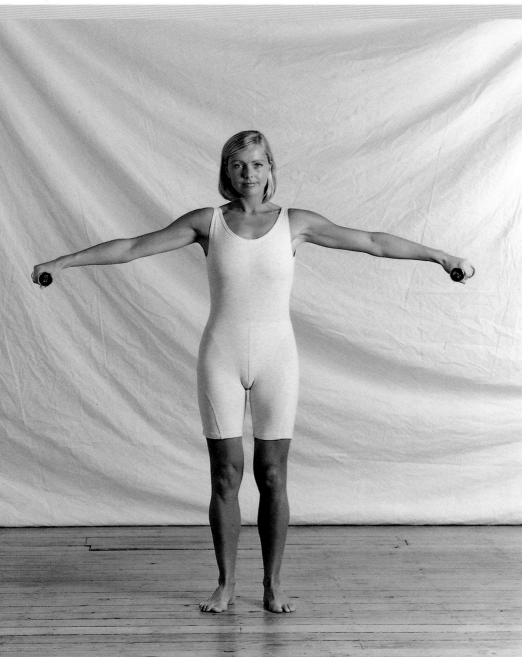

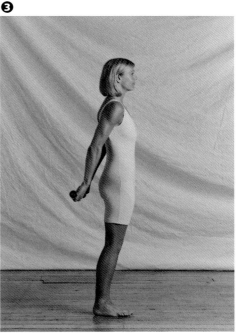

Raise and press

Each stage of this exercise will work a different area of your shoulder muscles.

Begin standing with good posture. For the middle of your shoulders, start with your arms by your side and your palms turned in toward your thighs. Raise your arms out to the side, no higher than shoulder level (1), then lower them.

For the front of your shoulders, start with your arms by your side and your palms facing back. Slowly lift your arms out in front of you to the level of your shoulders, keeping your palms facing down (2), then, just as slowly, lower them.

The last variation targets the back of your shoulders. Place your arms behind your back, resting the back of your hands on your buttocks. Slowly raise your arms behind you as far as they will go (3), and then gradually lower your arms back to the starting position. Make sure that your torso remains stable and upright and that you do not lean forward or roll your shoulders as you raise your arms.

To enhance any of these exercises, you can use weights, increasing the size as you grow stronger.

Biceps and triceps

Working in opposition, the biceps and the triceps are the main muscles in the upper arms. The biceps allow you to lift your arms in front of you, bend your elbows, and turn your palms up and down. Because they are used so frequently, they are often stronger than other upper body muscles. In most people, they are also stronger than the triceps, which lower your arms and straighten your elbows.

When you exercise your arms, you want to aim for increased strength and balance. As your arms become stronger, many day-to-day tasks, from carrying bags to working at a computer, will become easier. As your triceps develop in line with your biceps, you will experience more ease and fluency in your movement.

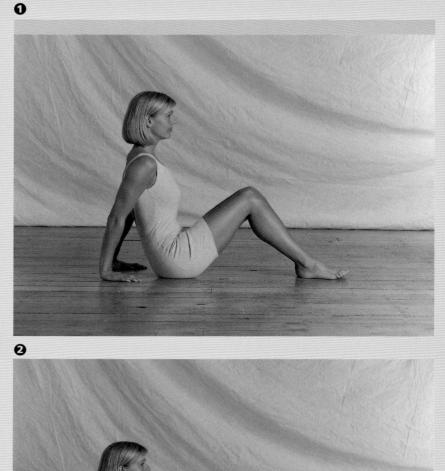

❶

❷

Tricep dips
This is the easiest version of the tricep dip. Begin by sitting on the floor with your knees bent and your feet flat on the floor. Place your hands on the floor behind you, shoulders' width apart, with your fingers facing forward: this will help you to stabilize your torso (1). By bending your elbows, ease your upper body halfway toward the floor (2), then straighten your arms, returning your upper body to the start position. Repeat 20 times.

①

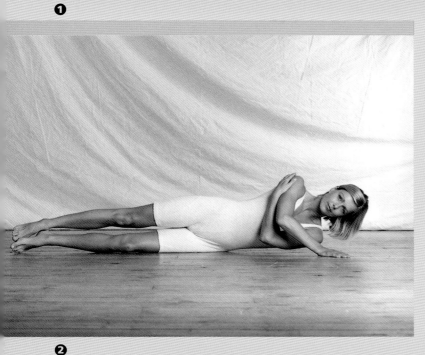

②

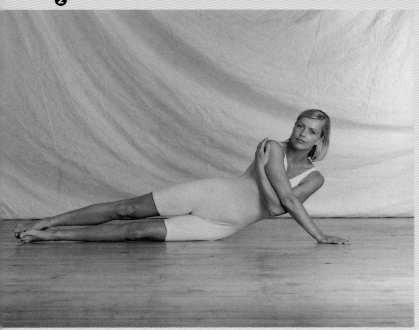

Tricep press-up

This is a very advanced exercise. Lie on your left side with both knees slightly bent, and place your right palm down on the floor in front of your chest for stability. Wrap your left arm under your right and place your left hand on top of your right shoulder (1). By pressing up with your right arm, raise your torso (2), then lower it by bending your elbow, making sure both movements are done slowly and with control. Stabilization is all-important in this exercise, so don't forget to pull in your abdominals and keep your back straight.

Bicep curl

Standing straight and strong, turn your palms away from you and make loose fists. Slowly bend your elbows and pull your forearm up to meet your biceps. Your wrists should be straight throughout. Gently lower your arms to the starting position before repeating 20 times. You can enhance this exercise by using weights, but make sure you do not rock your body as you raise and lower your arms. As a variation, you can turn your palms to face your thighs, and as you bend your elbows to raise your forearms, your thumbs head in toward your shoulders.

Upper back and lower back

Back pain, an all-too-common complaint these days, often results from weak back muscles and bad posture, particularly when sitting. The back muscles, working with the muscles of your chest and your abdomen, stabilize your torso and hold your body upright. Exercises that help to strengthen the back will help you to improve and maintain your posture and to avoid discomfort.

If you sit and stand with rounded shoulders, the muscles of your upper back are held in a continuously stretched position. In this case, you should emphasize exercises that strengthen this part of your body. It is in your lower back that you will feel the strain most.

Standing fly

Standing with your feet hips' distance apart, bend your elbows and raise them out to the sides in line with or just forward of your shoulders and just slightly lower than your shoulders (1). Pull your elbows behind your back as if you were trying to get them to touch (2). You should feel your shoulder blades squeeze together. Gently release your shoulder blades, allowing your elbows to return to the starting position, and repeat 12 to 20 times. Make sure you maintain good posture throughout the movement.

You can do the same movement more effectively by lying on the floor on your stomach, because you will be working against gravity. Without lifting your head, raise your elbows and pull them behind you, squeezing your shoulder blades together. Release and lower them to the floor, before repeating up to 20 times.

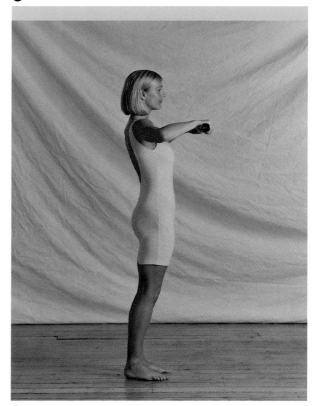

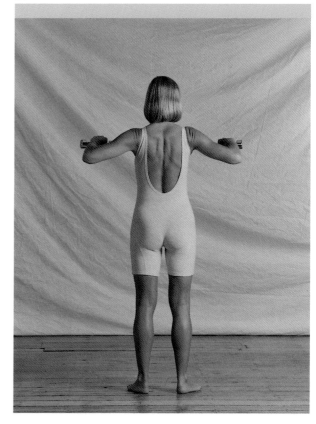

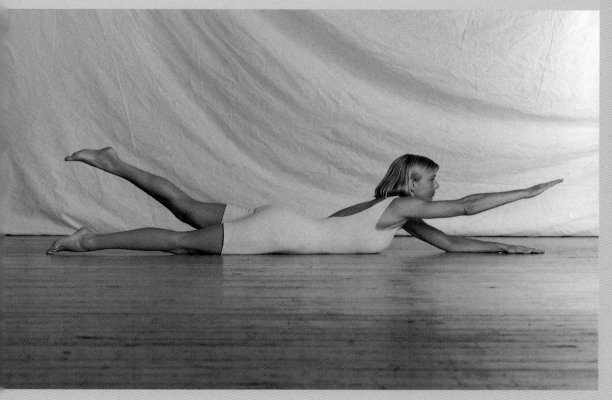

Opposite arm and leg lift

Lie on your stomach with your arms stretched out above your head. Keeping your hips and chest on the floor, lift your right arm and your left leg at the same time to the same height. Hold for as long as you are comfortable, aiming for 20 seconds. Lower the arm and leg to the floor, before repeating with your left arm and right leg.

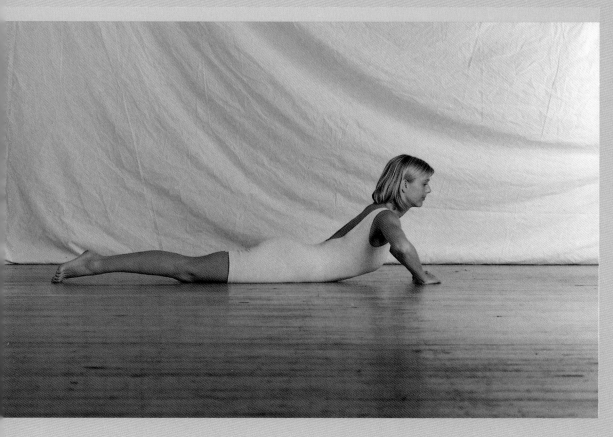

Lower back extension

Lying on your stomach with your hands under your chin, keep your hipbones and your feet on the floor as you press through your arms and lift your upper body off the floor as if it were one solid unit: visualize your spine as a metal rod that extends through your neck to the top of your head, so your head remains in a natural position. Although you should feel a pull along your back, you should not feel any discomfort. Use your arms for support as you lower your body back to the floor.

As an advanced variation, you can place your hands lightly on the small of your back or on your buttocks.

Chest

Much of our day-to-day movement is done to the front of our bodies. Think about the actions involved in pushing a shopping cart, working at a computer, or picking up an object from the floor or from a table.

To counteract the effects of the dominance of the front of the body, it is important to stretch out the chest muscles. At the same time, a strong and supple chest area helps to promote good posture, because it will prevent the shoulders from rolling

and the upper back from rounding both during exercise and other activity and at rest.

Since the front of the body tends to be stronger than the back, any exercises done for the chest should be complemented by upper back exercises (see pages 62–3) to develop a balanced torso.

As always, begin by working gently, especially if you have not done much work on your chest and upper back in the past.

❶
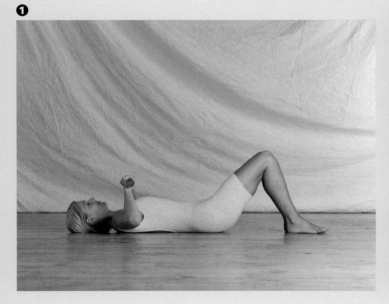

❷
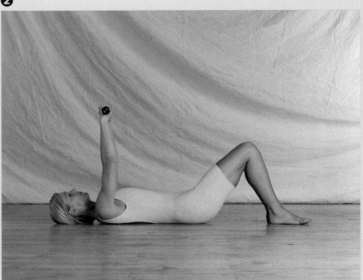

Chest press
Lie on your back with your arms straight out to the side, your knees bent, and your feet on the floor, and bend your elbows so your knuckles face the ceiling, trying to keep your upper arms in contact with the floor (1). Raise your elbows off the floor and straighten your arms toward the ceiling (2), then gently lower your arms, bending your elbows until they are again in contact with the floor. With practice, you can add weights to this exercise, increasing their size as you grow stronger.

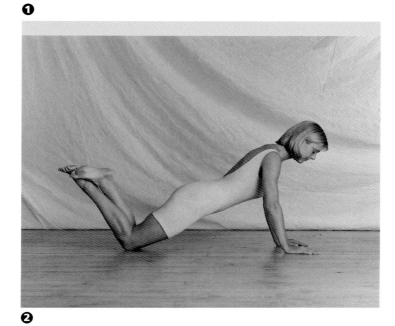

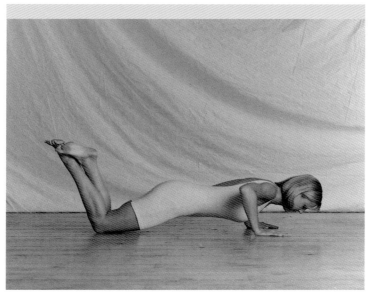

Press-up

On all fours, with your knees hips' width apart and your arms shoulders' width apart, lift your feet, cross your ankles, and lean forward, creating a straight line of your body from your knees to your ears (1). This line should be held as you slowly lower your body toward the floor by bending your elbows (2), then raise it slowly as you straighten them.

If you find this difficult, you can try the "box" press-up. Kneel on all fours, keeping your hips over your knees and your shoulders over your elbows and wrists. Bend your elbows and lower your chest toward the floor. Your nose is likely to touch the floor before your chest does. Stabilize your torso so your lower back does not sag, and keep your neck in alignment with your spine.

Torso

These gentle stretches will complement the strength moves you have done to work your upper and lower back, your chest, and your abdominals.

Strength exercises involve repeated contractions of the muscles. This means that they can cause the muscles to shorten, but complementary stretches will reverse that effect. They will help you to remain supple even as you are becoming stronger. Gently stretching your muscles after exertion will also help you to relax before moving to the next stage.

❶

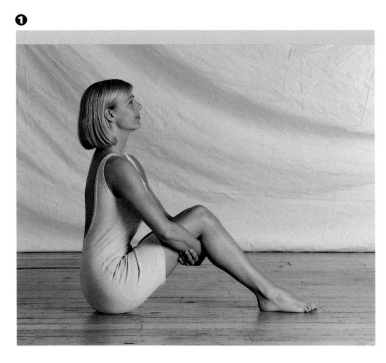

❷

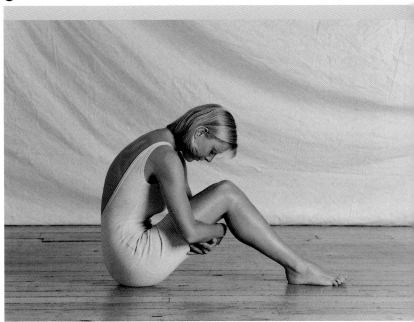

Crossed-arm back stretch

Sit on the floor with your knees bent and your feet on the floor. Wrap your arms under your knees, clasping your elbows (1). As you pull your abdominals in, lift and expand your back by separating your shoulder blades (2). Keep your arms clasped, using the resistance to enhance the stretch. Hold this stretch for around 20 seconds, then release and relax.

1

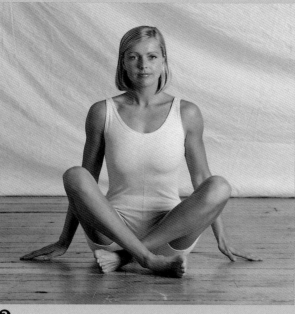

Sitting torso stretch

Sitting on the floor cross-legged, or in any other comfortable position (1), place your right hand on the floor to your right side for support, and reach your left arm overhead, feeling the stretch down the left side of your body (2). Hold this stretch for 20 seconds before relaxing, then switching sides.

2

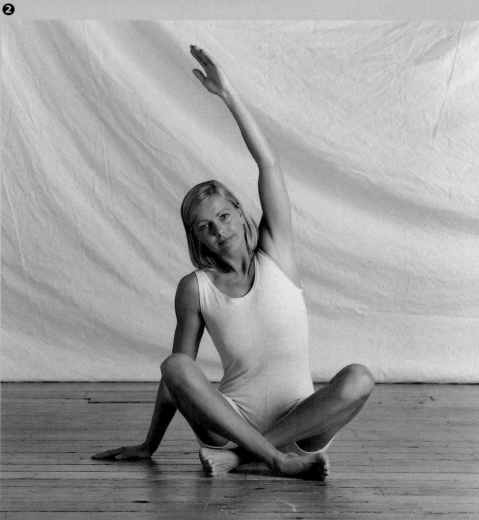

Abdominals

These types of abdominal exercise work the muscles safely but intensively. When you begin, do as many repetitions as you can manage, but remember, you are aiming for at least 20.

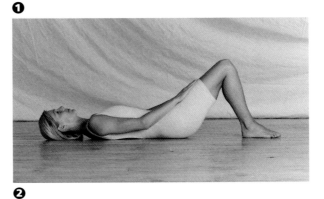

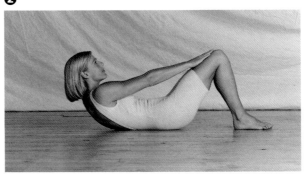

Curl-up

Lie on your back with your knees bent and your feet on the floor. Place your hands on your thighs (1). Pull your stomach muscles to close the gap between your back and the floor, then contract your stomach muscles so that your upper back, shoulders, and head lift (2). With control, lower your upper body toward the floor and, just before you get to a position where you feel you can relax, immediately repeat the sequence. Your chin should be in a natural position.

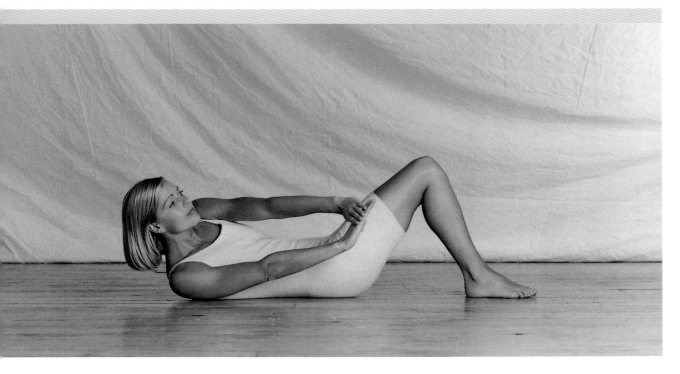

Oblique curl

This exercise is similar to the curl-up, but as you contract your abdominals, lift your left shoulder up and over toward your right hip, keeping your right shoulder on the floor. Slowly release your abdominals to lower your left shoulder to the floor. Your head and neck should remain in a natural position throughout. As a variation, you can place your right heel on your left thigh, and as you contract your abdominals, you should lift your left shoulder over toward your right knee.

❶

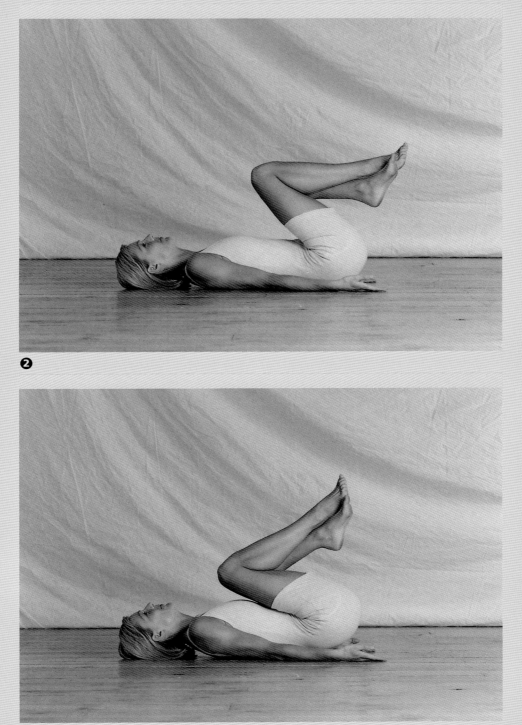

❷

Reverse curl

Lying on your back with your arms by your side and your palms turned up, bring both knees toward your chest, allowing your lower back to press into the floor. Cross your ankles and keep your heels close to your buttocks (1). As you contract your abdominals, your hips will lift up and forward and your knees will move toward your shoulders (2). Release in a slow, controlled manner, and repeat.

Legs

When exercising, it is easy to forget your lower legs, ankles, and feet. But wearing restrictive shoes can make this area of your body very tense and tight, so it is important to stretch from time to time. Also, the muscles in this region absorb a lot of the stress of walking, jumping, and running, and they will be more resilient when they are stronger and more supple.

Calf raises
Standing with your feet hips' width apart, using a wall or a chair for support, lift your right leg off the floor, resting the foot on your left leg, and slowly raise and lower your left heel. Keep your knees slightly bent throughout the movement: as you bend your knees deeper, the effort is concentrated lower down the calf muscle.

If this is difficult, you can work with both feet on the floor, lifting both heels at once, until you grow stronger.

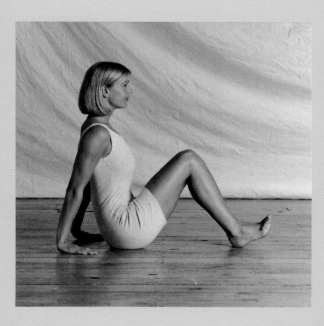

Toe taps
Sitting with bent knees and feet on the floor, lift and lower your toes and feet in a slow toe tap, keeping your heels on the floor. You can either work both feet at once, or alternate from right to left with single lifts. If you turn your feet in and out as you tap, you will be working with the muscles that run down the side of your legs to your ankles.

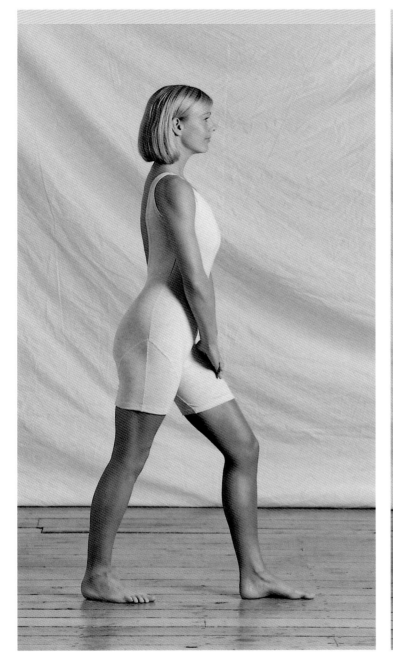

Calf stretch

Stand in a lunge position, with one foot in front of the other, and the knee of your front leg slightly bent and directly over your ankle. Move your rear leg farther back, keeping the heel of that foot on the floor, until you feel a stretch in your calf muscle. Hold for 30 seconds before repeating on the other leg.

If you bend the knee of your rear leg slightly, still keeping your heel on the floor, stepping in with your rear leg if you need to, you will feel a deeper stretch that works your lower calf.

Shin stretch

In a lunge position, lift your back foot and turn it under so the tops of your toes are resting on the floor. Bend the knee of your back leg and press the top of your foot toward the floor. You will feel the stretch along the top of your foot and in your shin. Hold for up to 30 seconds, then repeat on the other leg.

Routines

To save time and challenge yourself further, you can combine different exercises to devise a comprehensive workout covering your entire body. If you add together a hamstring curl and a tricep press-up, for example, you will be involving your whole body in dynamic movement.

By changing the combinations from time to time, you add variety to your exercise sessions. Think about changing your exercise routine every four to six weeks to keep yourself motivated – or you can have two different workouts that you alternate.

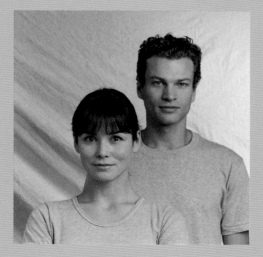

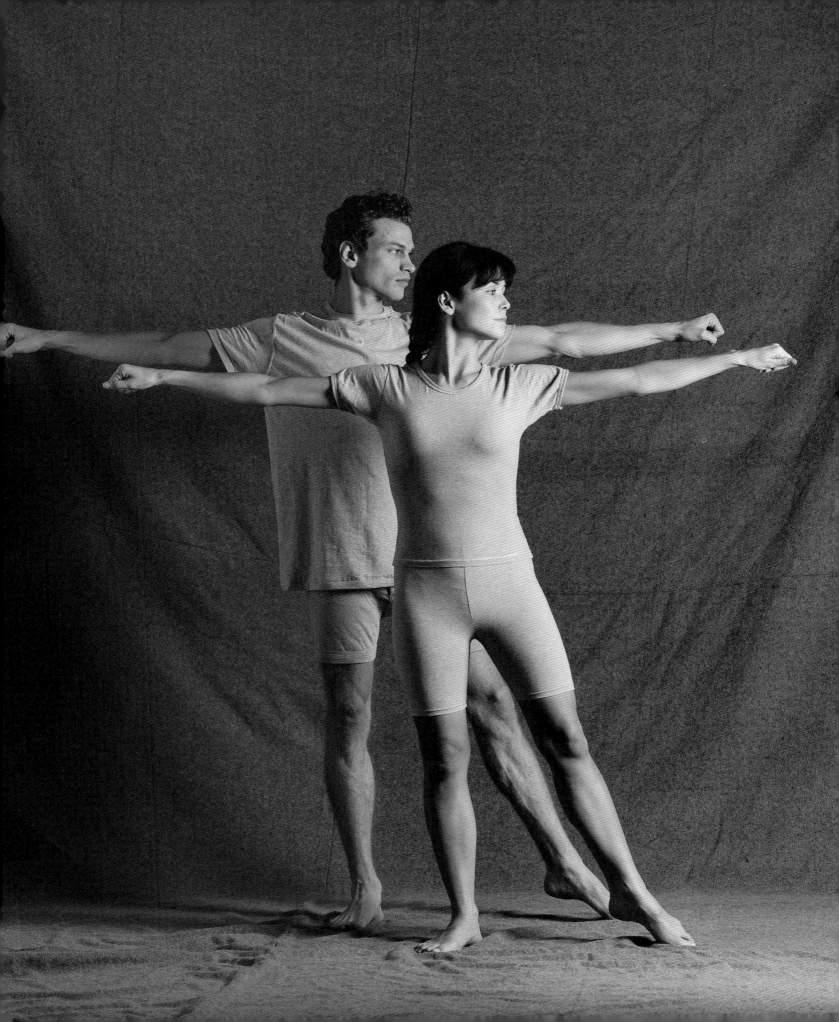

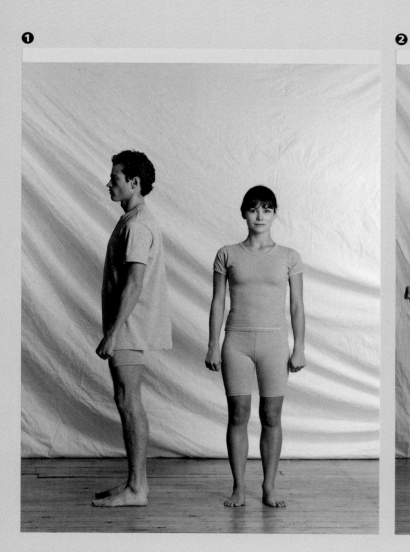

Squat and raise

Standing with your feet hips' width apart (1), bend your knees slowly to bring your hips down and back but no lower than your knees. As you squat, raise your arms out in front of you to shoulder height (2). The deeper you squat, the harder your legs will be working. As you stand up, lower your arms to your sides. Allow the movements to flow from one to the other.

If you want to make the exercise more challenging for your upper body, you can hold weights.

❶

❷

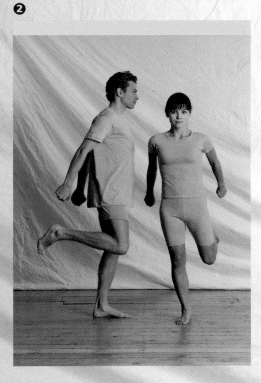

Tricep kickback

Begin with your feet wider than hips' width apart, your elbows bent close to your waist, and your hands in fists (1). Shifting your weight onto your right foot, lift your left foot behind you, like a standing hamstring curl. At the same time, straighten your elbows and push your arms behind your body (2). Return to the start and repeat on the other side.

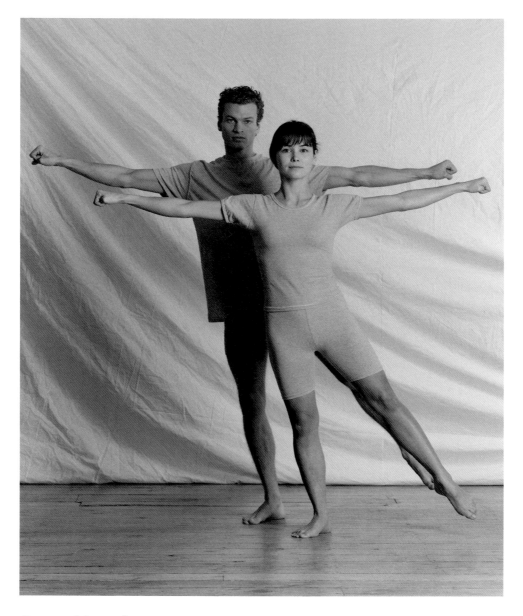

Arm and leg raise

Begin with your legs wider than hips' width apart and your knees bent. Straightening your right leg, raise your left leg out to the side at the same time as you raise both arms out to your sides to shoulder height. Return to the starting position, then repeat on the other side.

It is important to keep all the movements dynamic – when you return to the starting position, really punch your hands to the floor, and when you raise your leg to the side, make sure it is a strong movement. Work in a controlled fashion, making all your movements as big as you can.

❶

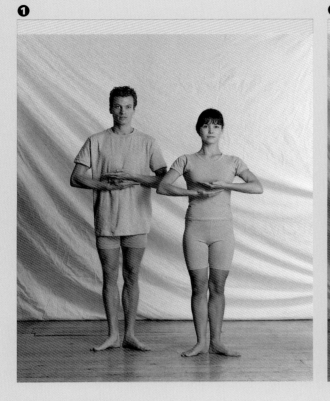

❷

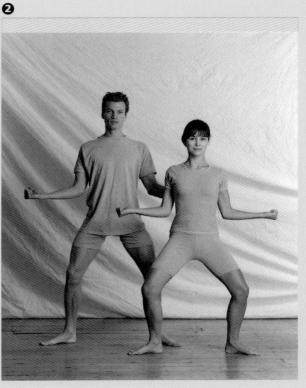

Cross and slide

Begin with your feet hips' width apart and slightly turned out, and your arms crossed in front of you (1). Step your legs apart to the left, bending your knees, at the same time as you open your arms, bringing your hands away from your body and your elbows in to contact with your waist (2). Slide your left foot back to the center, crossing your arms again.

You can increase the challenge in three ways: holding weights; making the squat deeper; and pressing your foot harder onto the floor as you slide.

❶

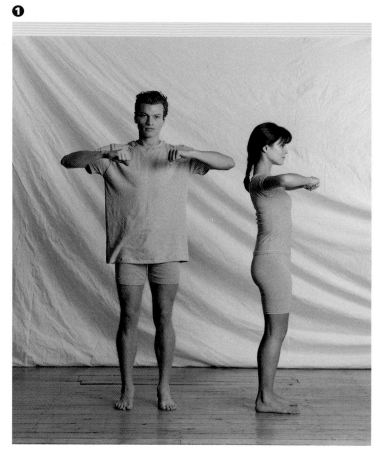

❷

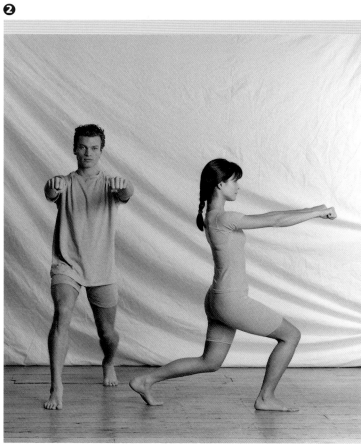

Chest press and forward lunge

Begin with your feet hips' width apart and your elbows bent and held out to the side at shoulder or chest level (1). As you step forward into a lunge, making sure you keep your front knee above your ankle, press your arms forward as if you were pushing something away (2). Bring your arms back toward your body as you step your feet back together.

You can challenge your muscles further by increasing the depth of your lunge or by holding weights.

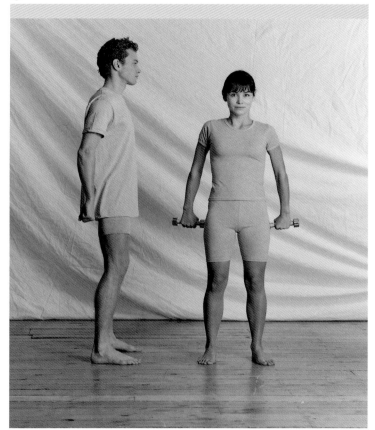

Press back and heel digs

Start with your feet hips' width apart and your arms resting on your buttocks, your hands clenched in loose fists (1). As you step forward with your right leg, touching your heel to the floor in front of you, push both arms straight back behind you (2). As your feet come together again, your arms should come back toward your body.

It might seem more natural to lift your arms in front of your body since your legs are moving forward, but making different demands on your body will keep your mind engaged and help you to improve your coordination.

You can increase the challenge by holding weights, or by bending your standing knee as you step the other leg forward.

Curl-up and reverse curl

By combining these two exercises, you will give your abdominal muscles a comprehensive workout.

For the curl-up, lie on your back with your knees bent and your feet on the floor, and place your hands on your thighs. Tighten your stomach muscles to close the gap between your back and the floor, then contract your stomach muscles to lift your upper back, shoulders, and head (1). With control, lower your upper body to the floor and, just before you get to a position where you feel you can relax, contract your stomach muscles again.

For the reverse curl, keep your hands by your side, your palms turned up. Bring your knees toward your chest, crossing your ankles, and allow your lower back to press into the floor. As you contract your abdominals, your hips will lift up and forward and your knees will move toward your shoulders (2). Release your abdominals in a slow, controlled manner.

For fun, devise different patterns of these two exercises in combination. For example, you could do eight curl-ups and eight reverse curls, then four of each, two of each, one of each. Or try doing them at the same time as an abdominal crunch, repeating this eight times.

As an advanced variation, you can hold your weights close to your ears or on your chest, if you are ready to increase your workload.

❶

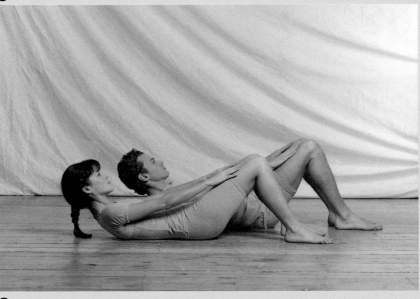

❷

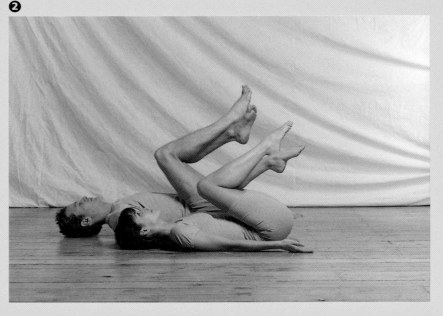

❶

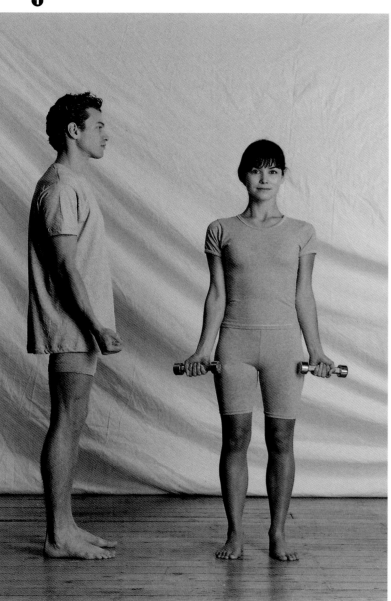

❷

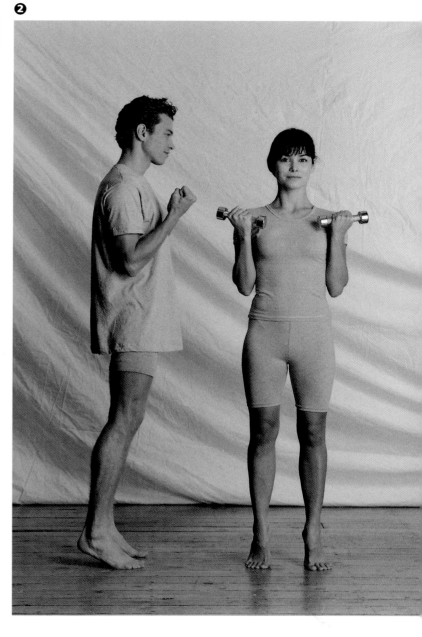

Bicep curl and calf raise

Begin with your feet hips' width apart, and your arms in front of your thighs with hands clenched in loose fists (1). As you raise yourself onto your toes to strengthen your calf muscles, bend your elbows and bring your palms up and in toward your shoulders (2). Lower your arms as you lower your heels. As a variation, you can use weights or lift one leg off the floor.

Abs and Back

The back and abdominal muscles are some of the toughest areas in the body, and even gentle toning will produce strong results. The most effective exercises for your abs and back are not the ones that make you sweat and strain. Work slowly and carefully, taking the time to listen to your body.

You may even want to repeat your favorite exercises each hour, particularly at first. This will make you more aware of your posture and improve the endurance of those muscles that hold you upright against gravity. Success – improvement in your posture and relief of any back aches and pains – will be quicker if you integrate the Core Exercises with some of the exercises from the Total Body Workout section. For best results, do the exercises little and often every day. A total of 10 minutes' exercise three to four times a day is ideal.

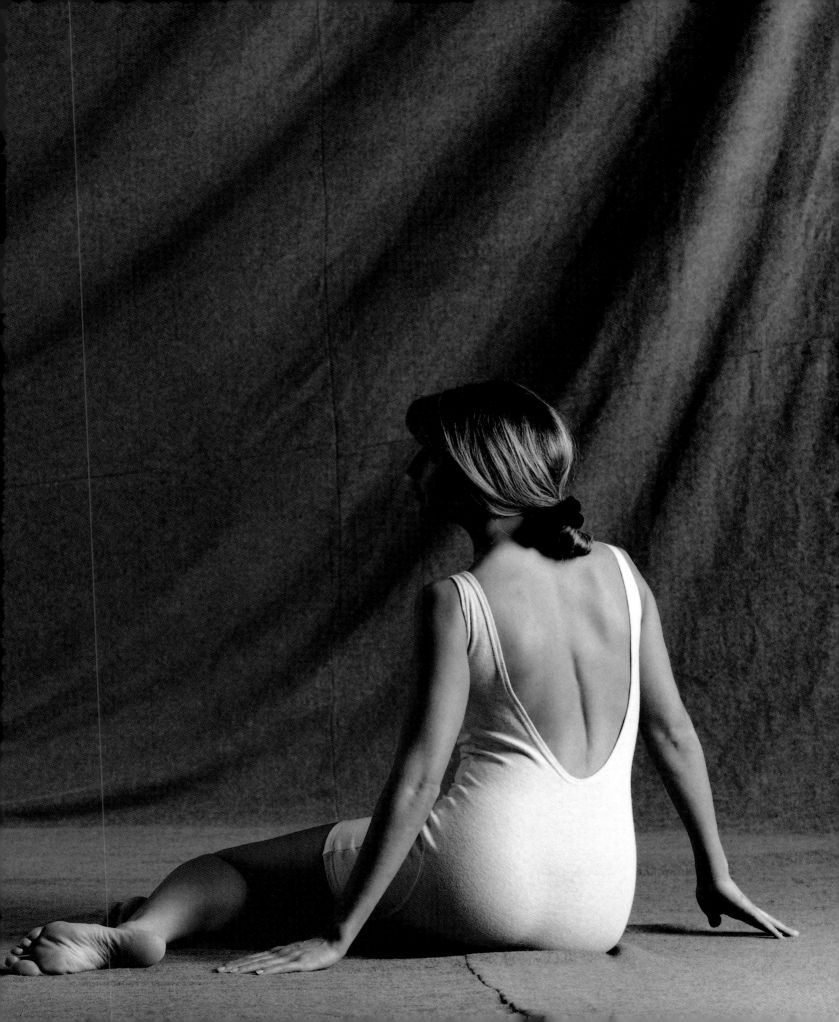

Back to basics:
posture

Take some time to remember the basics. If you treat your back without respect, sitting badly and straining as you lift heavy objects, there is a good chance you will pay the price. However, by remembering a few simple rules and doing a few easy exercises every day, your back will not only stay supple and relaxed, but your body will look great. And the really good news is that it couldn't be easier.

Nearly every movement you make – sitting down in a chair, walking to the front door, bending down to tie your shoe or to turn on the TV – involves your back in one way or another. Despite this, far too many of us take the workings of the back, and particularly the spine, for granted.

The back is also the key to a healthy posture. Posture is one of the main means by which we present ourselves to the world. For example, a depressed person will often appear bent or slouched, while a captain of industry will demand respect and obedience by puffing out his chest and holding his back ram-rod straight. An older actress will tell you that she can carry on playing youthful parts on stage by keeping her back supple, because the hunched back is perhaps the single biggest sign of ageing.

At the same time, posture is very closely linked to our emotional state, as well as our physical one. Our emotional state has two components: one is purely mental, and the other is physiological, and these two interact. The mind may instruct the body to respond in a particular way: for example, when we feel emotional pain, we often contract our body as if to protect it from harm. However, the mind also analyzes the state of the body and draws conclusions: if we sit and stand in a slouched position, the mind may interpret this as insecurity. Therefore, as you improve your posture, you will begin to feel more dynamic and more secure – this is why working on your back is such a rewarding experience.

A healthy posture not only looks and feels positive, but it also allows the body to function in an optimal way. Unfortunately there is much bad advice available when it comes to physical posture, and it is easy to forget that a healthy posture is the most natural thing in the world. Remember this as you work through the routines in this book.

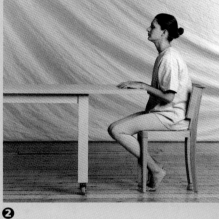

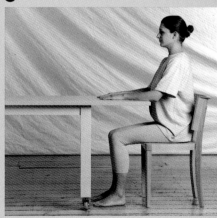

Sitting

Sitting slouched, with your chin jutting out, strains your back (1). To sit correctly (2), ensure that the height of your chair and desk are adjusted to your body size. Your feet should be flat on the floor, with your thighs not quite parallel to the floor. Your forearms should be parallel to your work surface.

The best way to understand how relaxed and resourceful the physical body can be is to look at the body of a child. A young child's back is long and straight, yet it is still relaxed. The head is balanced at the top of the spine without any unnecessary tension. Obviously everyone will lose some flexibility with age, but at the same time, many of us make physical activity harder than it needs to be. Much of the advice that is given here was second nature to us when we were children.

Sadly, we soon lose the child's easy, natural posture. Long hours are spent sitting in front of a computer screen or TV. We drive to the store instead of walking, and we stop playing sports once we leave school. All these factors, combined with the stress and strain of everyday living in the modern world, take their toll. Consequently you may find that your back feels stiffer than it used to, or in some cases you may find that the combination of poor posture and inactivity has led to spinal pain and muscular injury.

Think about your normal position when you sit. Do you slouch, with your chest concave and your bottom toward the front of the chair? This puts undue stress on the spinal disks and ligaments, and your back muscles and abdominals cannot support the spine. And if your head is thrust forward, this puts strain on your upper neck, often resulting in arm pains and headaches. A correct sitting posture will not create any unnecessary tension in the body. However, it is not a relaxed state either. Your lower back muscles should be working to keep your spine erect.

When you sit or stand with incorrect posture, you also restrict your breathing. The lungs have no muscles of their own: they take in air as they respond to changes in the size of the chest cavity created by movements of the muscles around the ribs, the back, and the abdomen. If you are slouched, the amount of space available for your lungs to expand is limited. As soon as the muscles in this part of the body are aligned and allowed to move freely, you will begin naturally to take deeper, more satisfying breaths.

To set yourself back on the road to that healthy state, you must begin to become more aware of how the back works. But remember, the aim is to release your back, allowing you to recognize its full potential. This cannot be forced or hurried. Simply telling yourself to

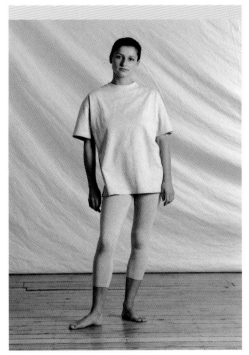

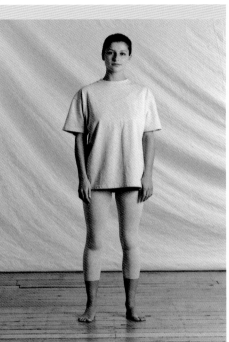

Standing

Standing with your weight over one hip, and your back and neck unaligned, not only looks unattractive, but can also lead to discomfort (1). When you are standing with good posture (2), your weight is evenly divided over both legs. Ideally, your whole body, from your ears through your shoulders, hips, and knees to your ankles, should be in alignment. Your knees and feet should be parallel and facing forward, with your weight balanced over your entire foot. Your abdominal muscles should be gently pulled in and up, supporting your lower back in its natural curve. Your shoulders should be parallel to the floor. Your head should be resting lightly on your neck, so your chin neither juts forward nor tucks down.

stand up straight or forcing your shoulders to relax will certainly do more harm than good. Excessive tension is the enemy of a healthy posture. However, as your muscles grow stronger and more accustomed to working together in a dynamic fashion, your posture will improve naturally.

Begin by trying this experiment. Sit on a firm chair and rest your hands on your thighs. Do nothing for a moment – just breathe easily and allow yourself to relax. Begin to picture your spine in your mind's eye (see the diagram on page 94 for reference). Take the index finger of your left hand and rest it as far down toward the bottom of your spine as possible. This will be about the top of your buttocks. Then, take the index finger of your right hand and rest it as high up your spine as possible. This will be just beneath the back of your skull between your ears. The distance from one finger to the other is the length of your spine. Long, isn't it?

Keeping your fingers where they are, experiment by moving your back in various ways. Slouch as much as possible, then sit up straight. Bend sideways or try to move only isolated parts of the spine. Notice whether different positions have any effect on your breathing. This will help you become more aware of the range of movement of which your spine is capable, and the more you become aware of this, the more that range of movement will increase.

By doing the exercises in this book, you will learn to be more aware of your posture. In addition, as your abdominal and back muscles grow stronger, your posture will improve without your making any conscious effort.

As you work through this book, then, you will begin to feel the benefits of having a stronger and more supple back and torso. You will feel taller, looking life straight in the eye.

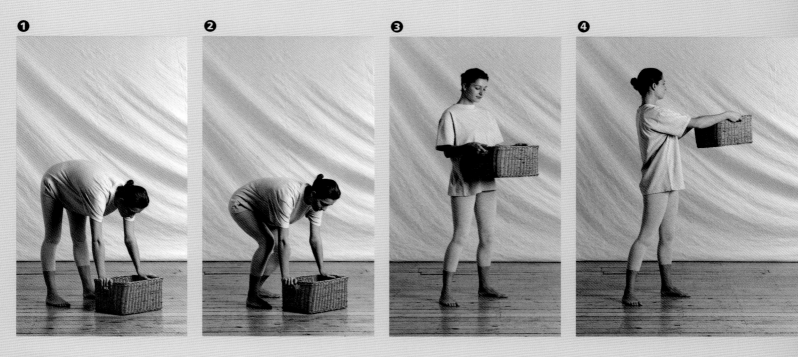

① ② ③ ④

Lifting

Lifting heavy objects with your knees locked straight and bending from the waist can lead to serious injury (1). Good lifting technique (2) means getting close to the object you are about to lift and bending your knees rather than your back. Feet should be wide apart to give you a good base of support. Always lift with your knees bent, keeping your back straight. It may be safer to "pre-set" your abs, tensing your lower abdominal muscles and lifting the object as you breathe out. When you are carrying heavy objects, keep them close to your body, to avoid strain on your shoulders, but do not lean backward (3). Do not twist your body as you are lifting – this combination of bending and twisting is responsible for more spinal injuries than any other form of movement. Rather, turn your body once you are standing straight (4). If you are going to be doing heavy lifting or other physical work, do a few warm-up exercises first.

Body facts

The human body is an intricate construction, with an amazing range of movement. Even the simplest movement is the result of a complex interaction of bone, muscle, connective tissue, and nervous system.

The spine, in particular, is a triumph of natural engineering. It consists of 24 oddly-shaped bones, formed so as to allow a remarkable range of movement – as long as the supporting muscles, in the back and abdomen, are strong and supple.

In order to improve the condition of your abs and back, you should understand the ways in which the muscles work together.

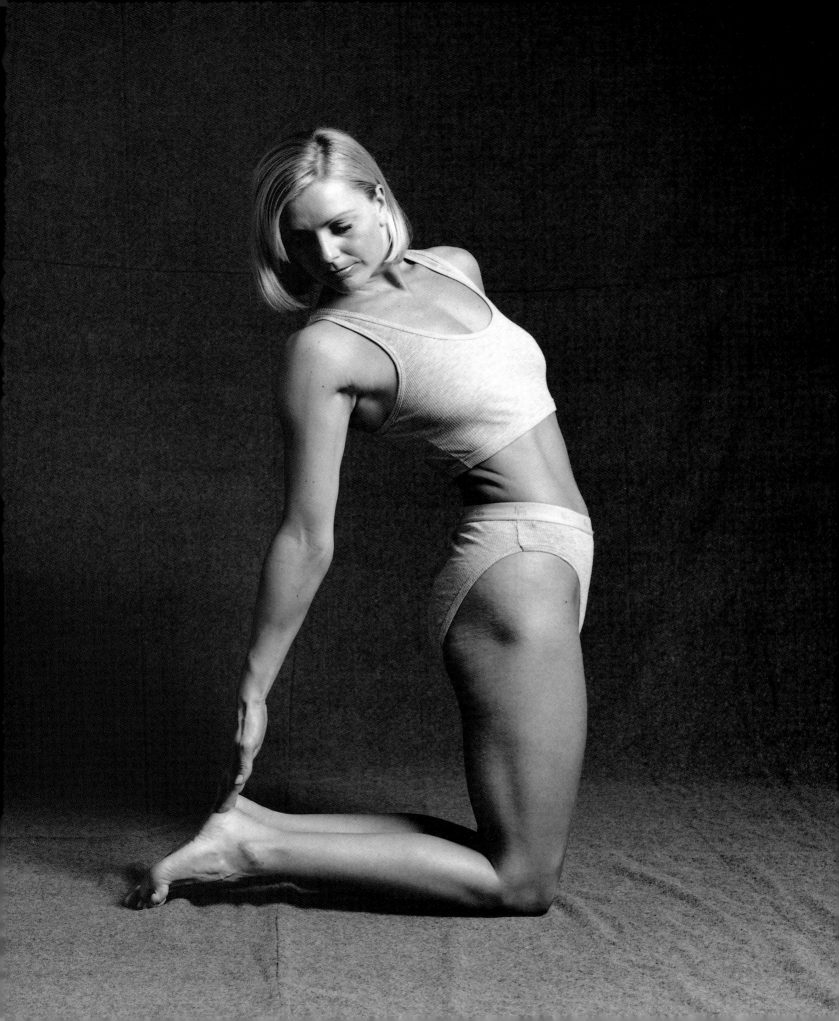

Body facts: abs and back

The torso – the back, abdomen, and chest – is the platform around which the arms and legs move. The trunk must be stable enough to support this movement and to stand upright, but it must also allow a wide range of motion, so you can bend forward and reach up and backward.

The spinal column is the foundation for the muscles of the back and neck. The vertebrae have different shapes and sizes depending on which part of the spine they come from. Those making up the lower back have wide, thick bodies, so they can cope with the forces coming down from the arms and upper back. The lower spine is designed to move backward and forward.

The 12 vertebrae that make up the mid-back, or thoracic spine, have special features to allow more twisting, or rotation, to occur. They also form joints with the ribs, which pass from the sides of the thoracic vertebrae around to the front of the chest where they form more joints with the chest bone. The neck is above the thoracic spine. It is designed to allow a great amount of movement and flexibility in all directions.

The pelvis is the basin on which the spinal column sits, and it connects the trunk to the legs. The stability of the pelvis allows the spine and legs to transmit forces through it.

The muscles that pass around the spine are responsible for both the dynamic stability of the spine and its movement. Each muscle has a specific function, and they all work in partnership to hold the body upright against gravity and to allow complex movements.

The muscles that aid the dynamic stability in the spine are deep muscles, lying very close to the disks and the vertebral bodies. Some pass over just one joint, but others may pass five or six different vertebral levels, with attachments to each vertebra. The muscles closer to the surface are moving muscles. Further muscles around the mid-back fix the shoulder blades to the spine and are responsible for both the mobility of the shoulders and arms.

The muscles at the front of the chest work in opposition to the back muscles to keep the spinal cord balanced. If there were no muscles at the front of the chest, the muscles of the back would pull the spinal cord backward.

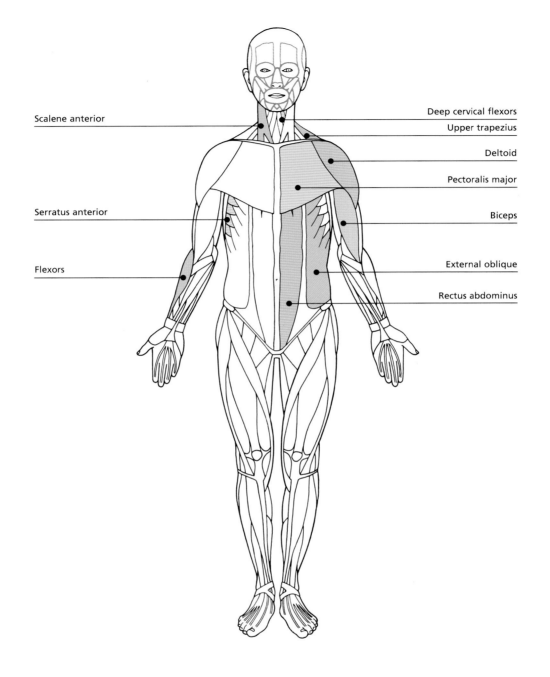

Scalene anterior

Deep cervical flexors

Upper trapezius

Deltoid

Pectoralis major

Serratus anterior

Biceps

Flexors

External oblique

Rectus abdominus

Front of the body

The abdominals are a group of four different muscles. One, the rectus abdominus, runs upward on either side of the midline of the body, from the pubic bone to the ribs. Its rippled form is easy to see on lean, highly developed bodies. The other three abdominals are flat sheets, layered one on top of the other. Underneath the external oblique are the internal oblique and the transverse abdominus. The muscles of the chest and shoulders work in opposition to the upper back muscles. If the chest is tight, the shoulders and upper back will hunch.

The muscles of the lower back also cross the pelvis and literally anchor the spinal column to the pelvis. They are responsible for keeping the whole spine in a balanced position.

The abdominal muscles work in unison with the lower back muscles and the muscles around the pelvis to keep this main platform stable. The abdominal muscles closest to the surface act as movement muscles, bending the trunk forward. The deeper abdominal muscles stabilize the lower back.

The buttock muscles pass across the lower back and pelvis. They keep the hip and lower leg in alignment with the spinal column, and act as the main propulsive force of the body when walking or running. At the same level but to the front of the spine are the hip flexors. These originate from the front of the vertebrae and pass through the pelvis to exit onto the top of the leg. They bend the leg forward and stabilize the lower back.

Because of the way in which the muscles of the body interact, problems in one area of the back may cause discomfort in other parts of the body (see illustration, right).

Cervical spine
•neck pain
•headaches
•arm pain

Thoracic spine
•shoulder pain
•upper back pain
•neck pain

Lumbar spine
•lower back pain
•groin pain
•thigh/calf pain

Sacrum spine
•lower back pain
•leg pain

Listed on the left, under the relevant headings, are regions of the body in which discomfort can be caused by problems in particular areas of the spine.

The spine
The spine is made up of 24 vertebrae, which are like bony building blocks stacked on top of each other. They are linked by two projections of bone at the back of each vertebra, one facing up and one down. The point at which these projections connect is a facet joint, and this is where movement in the spine occurs. This movement is limited by the contour of the bones – when they contact each other, further movement is blocked. The vertebrae are separated from each other by disks. They act as shock absorbers for the forces going up and down the spine and as a base on which each vertebra can pivot.

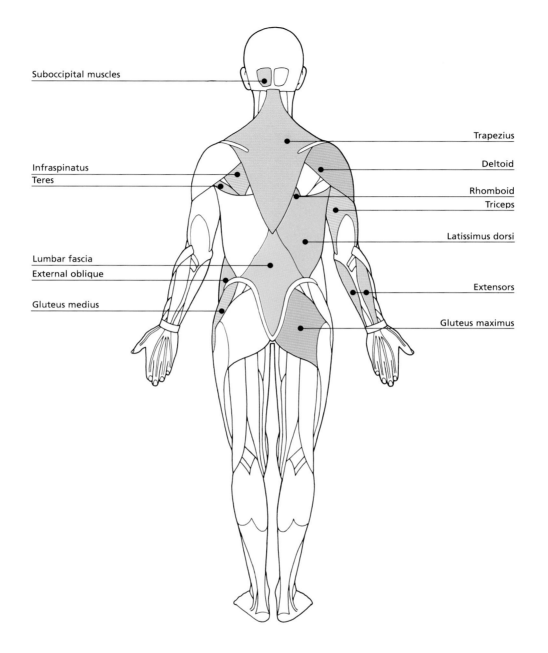

Suboccipital muscles

Infraspinatus
Teres

Lumbar fascia
External oblique

Gluteus medius

Trapezius

Deltoid

Rhomboid
Triceps

Latissimus dorsi

Extensors

Gluteus maximus

Back of the body

The muscles that aid the dynamic stability of the spine are very deep, lying close to the vertebrae. The muscles that are closer to the surface are the ones that are involved in movement. The external obliques are part of the abdominal group, which wrap nearly all the way around the body. The gluteus maximus is the major muscle of the buttocks: the condition of this muscle gives the buttocks their shape. The shoulder muscles, an intricate group, attach to the shoulder blades and to the collar bone. They work in opposition to the chest muscles.

Core exercises

If you spend a lot of time sitting during the day, the muscle groups running from the pelvis to the head will become progressively weaker with age. As these muscles struggle to hold your spine erect against the force of gravity, the joints of the spine become stiffer.

These core exercises will improve the strength of the supporting spinal muscles and the flexibility of the spine. Having a healthy spine will keep you looking and feeling younger and stronger. You will also feel healthier and more aware of your body when you do these exercises on a regular basis.

We all have different weak areas in our spines, so you can choose to focus on your own areas of discomfort. But if you are free of aches and pain, choose two or three exercises from each of the four sections. A few minutes' daily practice will allow you to maintain a strong and supple spine.

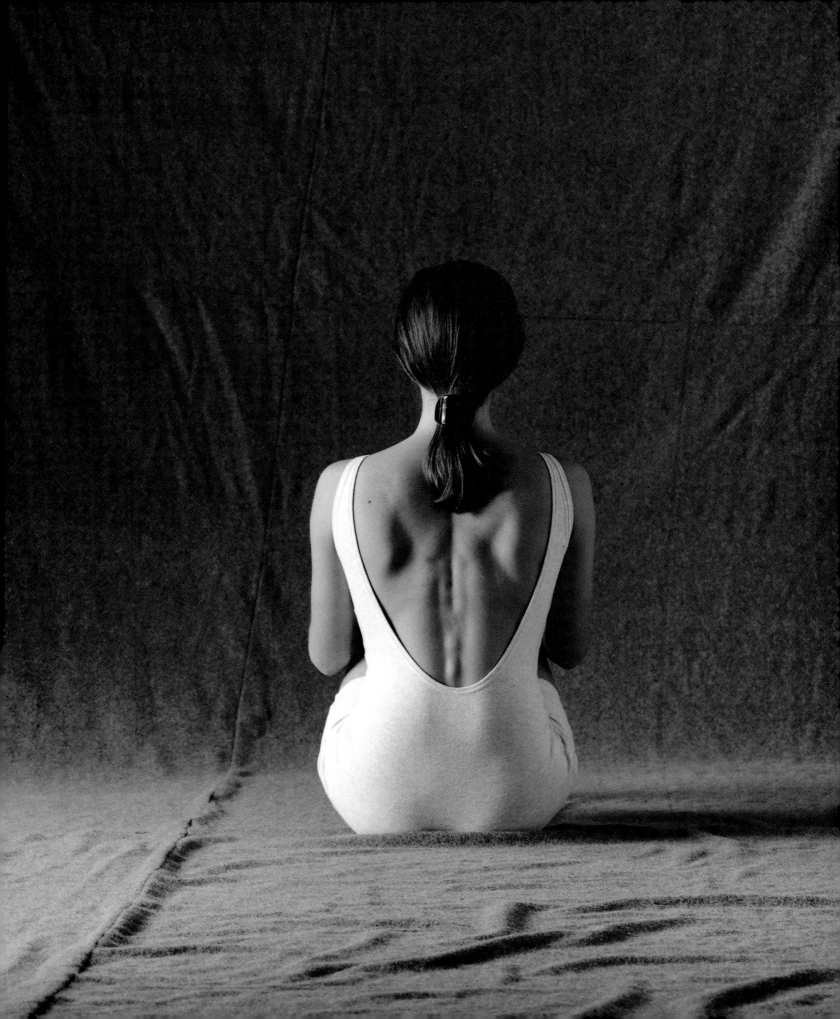

Head and neck

The group of muscles lying deep at the front of your neck is responsible for holding your head in good alignment on top of your spine and shoulders. If you sit with your head poking forward, these muscles weaken, and the muscles at the base of your skull tighten. When this happens, you feel an ache and stiffness at the top of your spine, and you may even experience headaches as the joints at the top of your neck take too much strain.

With exercises for the neck, it is essential to work gently. You should not feel any pain, and as soon as you feel you are losing control of what you are doing during an exercise, you must stop. Even if you can only do four or five repetitions of each exercise, this is enough. It is better to start slowly, gradually increasing the endurance of the muscles: if you push yourself too fast at the beginning, you can strain your neck muscles.

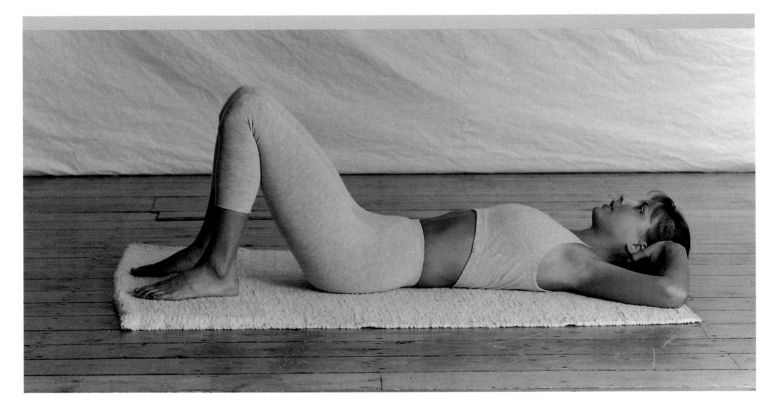

Neck lengthener

This exercise relaxes the muscles at the base of your skull, freeing them from tension caused by your daytime posture. It is also a good introduction to the other neck exercises.

Lying on your back (with your head on a pillow if you want), bend your knees and place your feet flat on the floor. Breathing slowly, deeply, and rhythmically, reach up with your hands and

place your fingertips into the hollow between your neck and your skull. Gently press your fingers into the muscle, and use your hands to lengthen your neck. As you do this, your chin should naturally tuck in. Hold this pressure firmly but without strain for 30 seconds to one minute. Repeat the exercise rhythmically for two to three minutes in total.

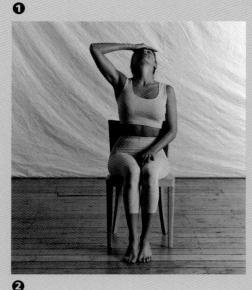

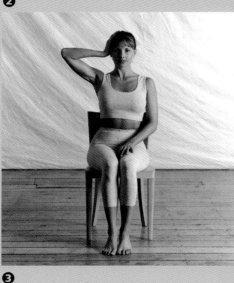

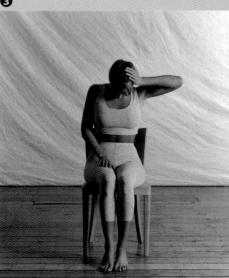

Head control series

This series of exercises is designed to strengthen the long muscles going from your shoulders to your neck and head. They are found at the front, back, and side of your neck.

Sitting tall, with your head balanced naturally on your neck, place both your hands on your forehead and apply pressure with your hands as if you were going to push your head backward. You should match this pressure from your hands with an equal pressure from the muscles around your neck, keeping your head in the mid-position – don't allow your hands to move your head. Start off gently, and gradually increase the pressure from your hands.

This exercise should be done gently and should be pain-free. You can vary the position of your head, applying the pressure to the front, back, and sides of your head, either with your head flopped forward, chin on your chest, or while looking up toward the ceiling, so your head is arching backward. For example, placing your hand on your forehead and tipping your head gently back, you can push forward with your head as you push lightly back with your hand (1). Or place your right hand on the right side of your head, just above your ear. Apply pressure with your hand, trying to push your head to your left shoulder (2). Again, don't let this movement happen: resist it with the muscles around your neck. You can do the same thing while your head is in a forward position (3).

Upper back

Your upper back stores a lot of tension, especially if you spend time sitting at a desk or working at a computer. In addition, when you feel stress, this part of your body tightens: just talking about being "uptight" can make your shoulders rise toward your ears.

The muscles of the upper back need to be both strong and supple: strong enough to contribute to the stability of the torso, and supple enough to allow the spine its full range of twisting movement, in order to prevent strain on the shoulder joints and the neck.

Some of these exercises will stretch the upper back and spine, and others will make the muscles around the upper back and shoulders work more efficiently. Decide which you are in need of most – more movement or more strength – and make your choice of exercises accordingly.

Even if you have a forward curve in this part of your back and you haven't been able to straighten up for some time, you will notice changes occurring quickly as you start to move in a healthier way.

❶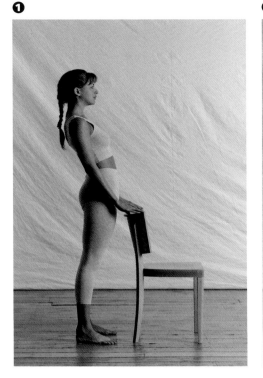

❷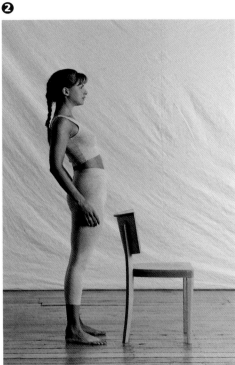

Shoulder shrug

Standing with your feet hips' width apart, your knees slightly bent, and your arms hanging by your side, lift up your chest a little and shake your shoulders and arms (1). Imagine that you are cold and your shoulders and arms are shivering. After doing this for 10 to 15 seconds, do slow, gentle shoulder shrugs, moving your shoulders backward. Lift your shoulders up toward your ears, and keep your shoulders high as you roll them backward (2), then relax your shoulders so that your hands drop further down toward your knees. Repeat this exercise six times.

Wall push

Stand facing the wall, with your feet about a foot (30 cm) away and balanced under your hips. Lift up your chest a little, tightening your buttocks. Bend your elbows and reach forward with your arms so your forearms rest against the wall – they should be parallel and shoulders' width apart (1).

Push into the wall with your forearms and maintain this pressure as you slowly slide your forearms up the wall about five inches (13 cm) (2). Keep your chest lifted as you slowly slide your arms back down the wall. Make sure you don't shrug your shoulders up toward your ears. Repeat this exercise six times.

This exercise works the muscles around your shoulder blades, and sometimes you may even feel a slight burn in this area.

❶

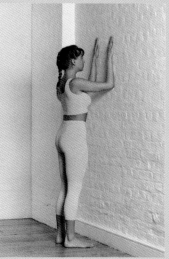

❷

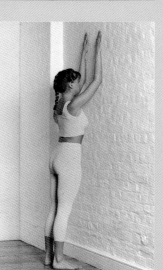

❶

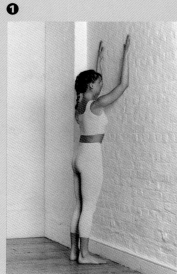

❷

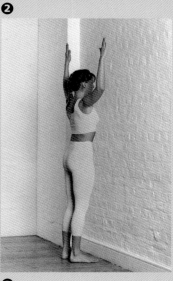

❸

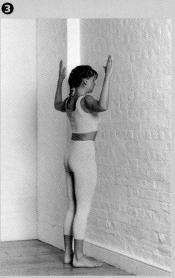

Wall push and drop

Stand facing the wall, with your feet about one foot (30 cm) away and balanced under your hips. Lift your chest a little and tighten your buttocks. Bend your elbows and reach forward with your arms so your forearms are resting against the wall, with your forearms wider than shoulders' width apart.

Slowly slide your forearms up the wall for five inches (13 cm), maintaining the pressure (1). Once you have reached this position, move your forearms a little way back from the wall (2), keeping your chest lifted high, your shoulder blades tucked down, and your elbows up. Now, slowly lower your arms back down (3). Repeat this exercise 10 times.

A slight burning feeling around the shoulder blades is normal and means you are working the correct muscles, but you should not feel pain.

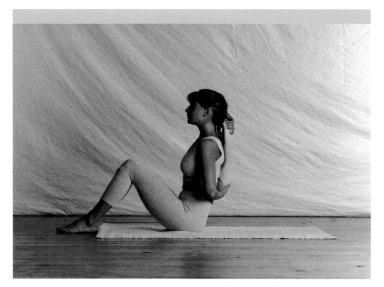

Towel stretch

Lie on your back (with your head resting on a pillow if you want), your knees bent, and your feet flat on the floor. Place a rolled towel beneath you along your spine, from the base of your neck to just below the bottom of your shoulder blades. You should feel balanced on the towel and not twisted to either side.

In this position, do nothing – just breathe deeply and allow your shoulders to relax over the rolled towel. You may feel some stretch around your shoulders or at the front of your chest. This is a good sign and means that the joints are gradually becoming more supple, and the tight muscles are stretching. Remain in this position for up to 10 minutes.

Consider it a relaxing time. It is best to do this exercise at the end of the day, but do not do it in bed, because you need to be resting on a firm surface to achieve the most benefit.

Bath stretch

This exercise stretches the nerve tissue in your spinal cord as it connects down your leg. It also stretches the joints between your ribs and the vertebrae in your upper back.

Sitting on the floor, with your knees slightly bent and a pillow or a rolled towel beneath them, cross your arms across your chest. Allow yourself to slouch and in this slouched position, twist your body to the left. Hold this stretch for 10 seconds, then repeat to the right. Do this exercise three or four times to each side. When you are more supple, you can remove the pillow and sit with your knees straight and your legs stretched out in front. However, if you experience an uncomfortable stretch in the backs of your legs or tingling in your feet, then this stretch is not for you.

Body spin

Sitting in a chair with your feet flat on the floor, your arms raised to shoulder level with your hands meeting in front of you, turn your head to the left, then follow with your shoulders. Stretch around as far as you can, as if you were straining to see something behind you. Hold this stretch for 10 seconds, then repeat on the opposite side. Do a total of three twists to each side.

Lower back strength

The muscles of your lower back play a crucial role in stabilizing the lower part of the spine and the pelvis. If they are working well, there will be very little strain to the joints and disks of your back, but when they are not, you will experience increased strain on your lower spine and, sooner or later, some back pain. This is because the muscles act to hold your spine up against gravity. They also work as shock absorbers, taking the body's weight as you walk or run.

These exercises must be repeated a minimum of 15 times each. Do the exercises slowly and think about the position of your lower back in relation to your pelvis and upper back. Try to visualize these muscles getting stronger as you do each repetition.

You should not feel any extra back pain either during the exercises or immediately after finishing them. With continued practice, you will note your posture improving and any back pain disappearing.

❶

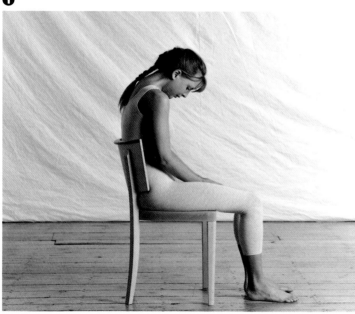

❷

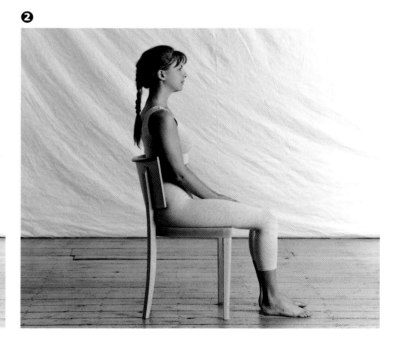

The extender
This is a great exercise to do whenever you are sitting down, and is also a warm-up for the other back strengthening exercises.

Sitting on a chair with a slouched posture, keep your feet flat on the floor (1). By squeezing your buttocks, you will feel that you are rising a little in your chair. Continuing to squeeze your buttocks, lift your chest, straightening up from the slouched position and feeling even taller, using your lower back muscles to raise your body (2). Hold for 20 seconds, then relax and repeat.

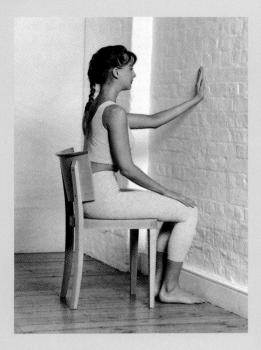

Strength push

Sit in a chair facing a wall, with your buttocks squeezed and your chest lifted, breathing easily from your lower chest. With your left arm, push your hand into the wall as if you were trying to push the wall away, but do not let any movement occur in your trunk or spine. The muscles of your lower back will be resisting the twisting movement that you are attempting by pushing the wall away. Hold this contraction for 15 seconds and then repeat with your right arm. Repeat four times on each side.

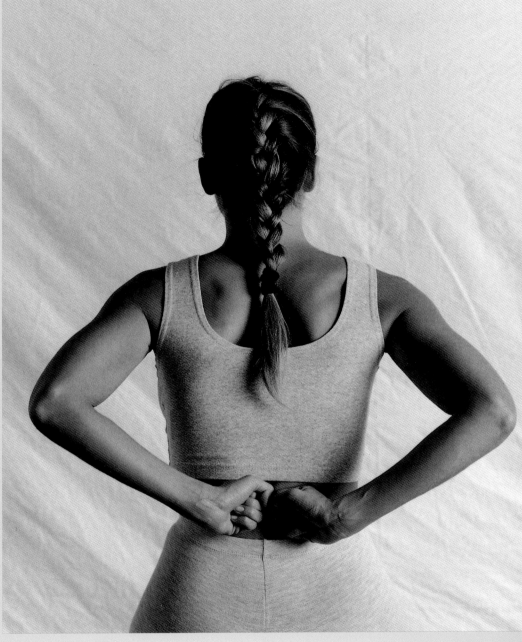

The back pump

Sitting in a tall position with your buttocks squeezed and your chest lifted, and breathing easily from your lower chest, rest your knuckles just on either side of your spine. Tighten your abdominal muscles, but don't hold your breath. As you do this, you should feel your muscles swelling underneath your thumbs. If you have a particular area of lower back pain, place your knuckles there; if you don't, move your knuckles up and down, working at different levels. Hold the muscle swell for 15 seconds, and repeat four or five times.

Lower back stretch

Most people will experience some stiffness in their lower back at some time, either with or without pain. This stiffness occurs when the muscles of the lower back are not working efficiently, causing strain. To avoid this, it is important to stretch out the muscles and joints of the lower back at the same time as you do strengthening exercises.

You should choose only three or four of these exercises to incorporate into your daily routine. It is good to feel a stretch in your lower back when you are performing these exercises, but if you feel any pain or discomfort, you should not push the exercise any further: just relax and breathe deeply, and the discomfort should pass.

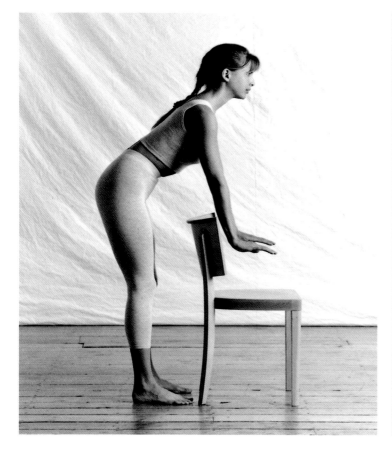

Waiter's bow
Stand behind a chair with your weight equally on both feet and your feet aligned under your hips. Squeeze your buttocks and hollow your lower abdominal muscles by contracting them before you begin any movement. Keeping your back straight, lean forward from the hips, slowly sliding your hands down the back of the chair and letting the chair guide your movement. When you have gone as low as you can, hold the stretch for 10 seconds before slowly returning to the standing position, keeping your back straight.

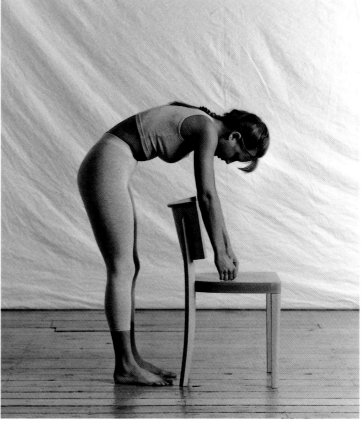

Puppet
Imagine yourself suspended by strings like a puppet. Think how it would feel if the strings supporting the top of your body broke.
Stand behind the back of the chair with your weight equally on both feet. Starting with your head, curl forward so your chin touches your chest, then continue the curling movement from your upper back down, slowly curling until you have gone as far as you can. At this point hold the stretch for 10 seconds. On the way back up, gently uncurl from your lower back to your upper back, then your neck and finally your head.

Chair twist

Stand facing a chair and place your left foot on the seat. Slowly bend forward, reaching inside your bent knee as you come forward. You will feel yourself twisting toward the right from your hips. Don't bounce as you do this exercise – slowly and smoothly allow your body to go as far as it can naturally. Repeat this exercise six times on each side.

Sciatic back stretch

This exercise will stretch the sciatic nerve, which runs from the base of your head to the back of your leg and foot. You should not experience tingling in your leg or pain in your back when you do this exercise.

Sit on a chair and slouch, allowing your chin to tuck onto your chest. Slowly straighten your left leg, flexing your foot. Stop as soon as you feel a gentle pull in the back of your leg. Hold this position for three seconds, then place your left foot back on the floor before returning to a tall sitting position. Repeat on the opposite leg. Do no more than two repetitions on each leg.

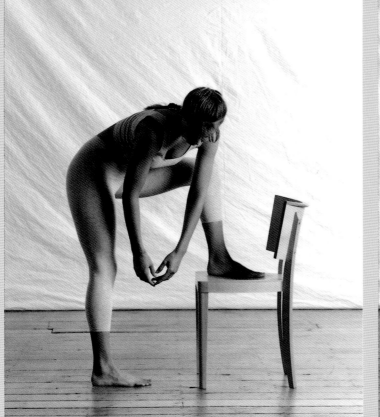

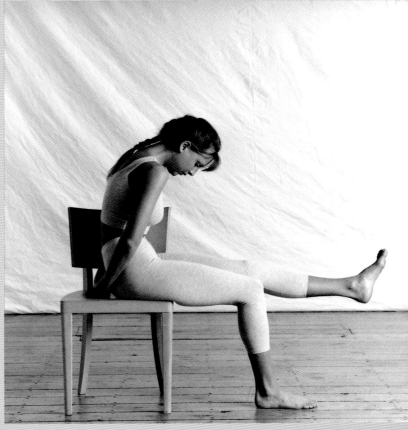

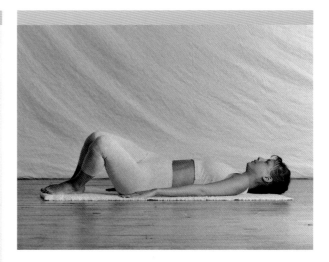

Back roll

Lie flat on your back with both knees bent, feet flat on the floor, and your arms by your sides. Slowly allow both of your legs to fall toward the right, stretching the left side of your back, until your right leg rests on the floor. Stop if you feel any discomfort in your lower back. Hold this position for six seconds, and repeat three times on each side.

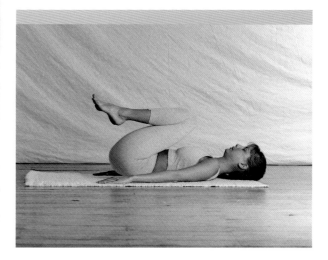

Double hip curl

Lying flat on your back, bring both your knees toward your chest and clasp them with your hands. Pull gently on your legs to help curl your knees up toward your chest. You should have rolled up into a ball. Hold this position for 20 seconds before relaxing to the floor. Repeat three times.

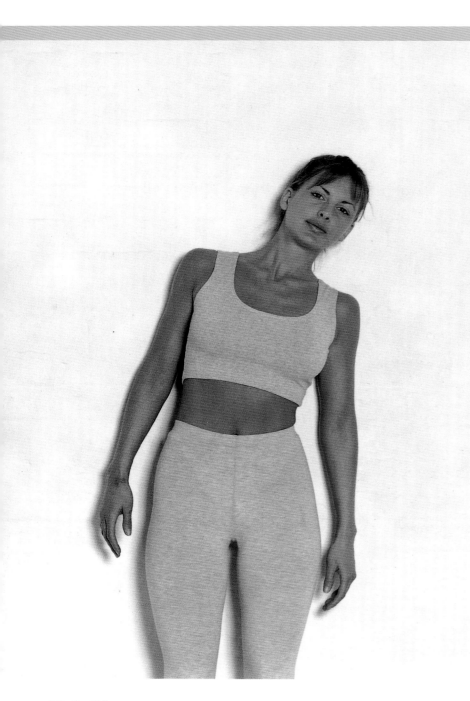

Wall slide

Stand with your back to a wall, leaning against it, with your feet two foot-lengths away and your knees slightly bent. Tighten your low abdominal muscles and flatten your lower back against the wall, imagining a brace holding your lower back flat against the wall. Slowly allow your left hand to reach down toward your left knee, bending your upper body to the side as you go. Reach as low as you can, holding the stretch for 10 seconds, before slowly sliding back to the starting position. Repeat six times on each side.

Hip curl

Lying flat on your back, bend your right leg up toward your chest, and reach down with your hands to clasp your knee. Lightly pull your knee in toward your chest, feeling a gentle stretch in the small of your back and right buttock. Hold this position for 20 seconds, before relaxing to the floor. Repeat three times on each leg.

Cobra

Lie face down on the floor with your weight through your forearms, elbows bent and under your shoulders. Pushing through your forearms, lift your head and chest high, and the small of your back will arch gently. Hold for 30 seconds, then relax back to the floor before repeating three times.

For a more advanced version of this stretch, place your hands underneath your shoulders as you lie face-down. Slowly lift your head and shoulders and then push through your hands to straighten your elbows (see picture). Your upper back should arch first, followed by your lower back. Keep the front of your hips on the floor. Stop as soon as you feel a stretch in your lower back, or if you cannot arch any further because of stiffness. Hold this position for 30 seconds and repeat three times. If you experience any lower back pain during this exercise, return to the basic stretch until you are more supple.

Abdominals

The abdominal muscles are essential in supporting the trunk. By strengthening them, you lessen your chances of lower back strain, because the abs and the lower back work in partnership.

Because the abs are a group of four different muscles, you have to do a variety of different kinds of exercises if you want to work them all. For example, twisting movements work the obliques at the side of the trunk, while crunches act on the muscles to the front of the abdomen.

With all these exercises, it is important to work slowly and carefully. Do not move to the more advanced exercises until you are strong and confident, and if you feel any lower back pain during one of the exercises, stop immediately and spend a few more sessions working on easier variations before trying that exercise again.

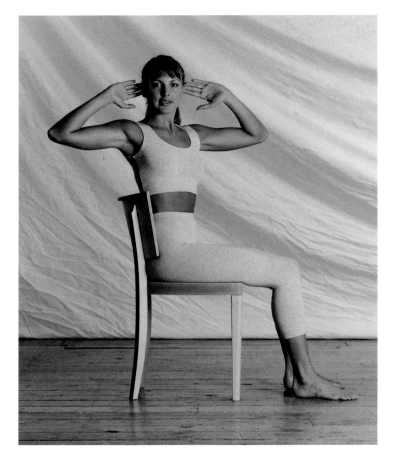

Seated twist
Sit on a firm chair, your feet flat on the floor, and rest your hands near your ears with your elbows pointing out. Twist so your left arm and elbow come across your body, without bending forward or tilting. You should feel your abdominals working, as well as a slight stretch in your upper back. Hold for a few seconds, before relaxing and repeating on the other side.

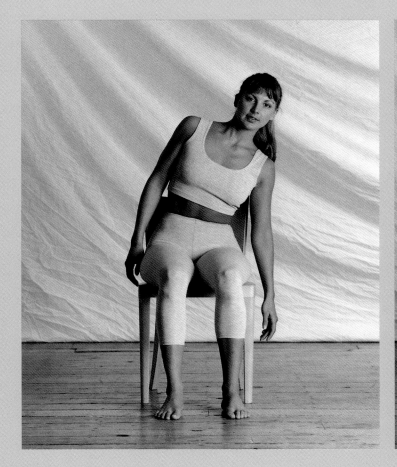

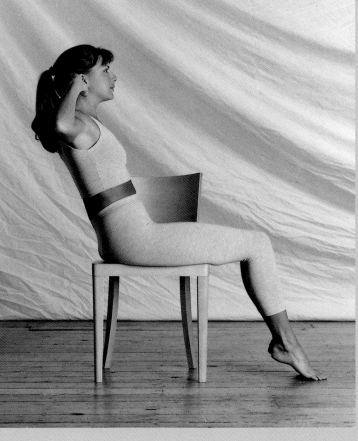

Side bend
Sit toward the edge of the seat of a firm chair, your feet flat on
the floor and your arms relaxed by your side. Without tilting
forward, bend to the left, lowering your left hand toward the
floor. Straighten up before lowering your body to the right.
Repeat 10 times on each side.

See saw
Sit on a firm chair, with your hands behind your head, elbows
out to the side, and your feet flat on the floor. Keep your back
straight as you slowly tilt forward from the waist, then straighten
up before tilting backward. Repeat 10 to 12 times, continuing to
move slowly and evenly. If you have any lower back pain, stop
and relax, and come back to this exercise a few weeks later.

Chair march

Sitting on a firm chair with your feet flat on the floor, lean backward, keeping your back straight. Slowly raise one leg, keeping your foot and knee in line with your hip, and lower it before repeating with the other leg. Repeat 10 times on each leg. To make this exercise more challenging, you can lean back further or lift your leg higher.

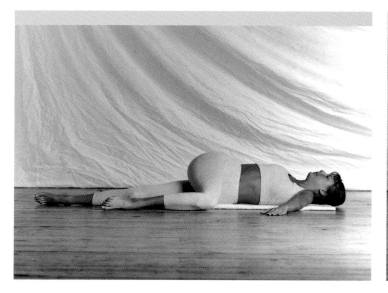

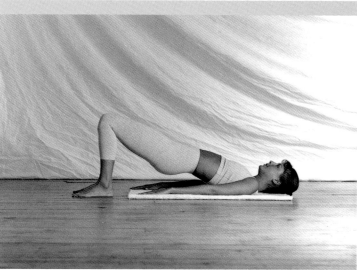

Lying leg roll

This is a good stretch for the lower back and back of the thighs. Lie on your back, with both legs straight, and your arms gently stretched out at shoulder level and resting on the floor, so your body makes a "T" shape. Bend your right knee and and lift your right leg up and over your body to roll toward the left. Hold this position for six seconds, before relaxing and repeating three times on each side.

Abdominal tilt

Lie on your back on the floor with your knees bent and your feet, knees, and hips in line with each other. Keeping your feet and shoulders still and squeezing your buttocks, raise your pelvis and lower back into the air in one slow, controlled motion, until the front of your body, from your thighs through your abs and chest, makes a flat plane, then lower yourself back slowly to the ground. Repeat 10 times.

Basic crunch

Lying on your back with your knees bent and your feet flat on the floor, and your hands resting by your ears, tighten your lower abdominal muscles and, keeping your lower back stable and on the floor, curl up slowly, head and upper back first, until you reach the limit of your movement. Don't lead from your head – make sure you keep your neck aligned with your spine, working from your abdominals. Relax down to the floor, then repeat 10 times in total.

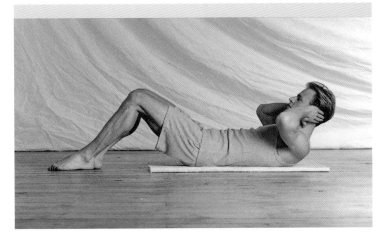

Side-lying oblique

This exercise works your obliques on the side of your trunk. It will help to trim your waist and give more support to your spine. Begin by lying on your left side with your knees bent and in line with your hips, then turn your upper body so your head and shoulders are flat on the floor, and rest your hands by your ears. Crunch up, moving first from the head then your upper chest, middle chest, and finally your lower back, then relax down, reversing the process, moving slowly and smoothly throughout. Repeat 10 times on each side.

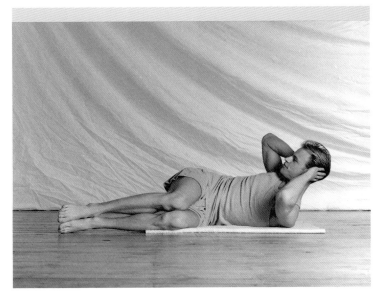

Side-bending toe reach

Lying on your back with your knees bent and feet flat, lift your head and shoulders slowly off the floor and bend down and sideways so your left hand reaches toward your left foot. Return to the center, keeping your head and shoulders off the floor, then bend toward the right side. Don't try to stretch too far – it is only a small movement. Repeat 10 times on each side.

High toe reach

This is an advanced exercise, which you should only try once you have mastered the other abs exercises.

Lie on your back with your feet pointing toward the ceiling, with your ankles crossed, your knees relaxed and slightly bent, and your left arm under your head. Slowly lift your head and shoulders from the floor and reach to your feet with your right hand. Return to the floor before repeating on the other side. Repeat as many times as you can on each side.

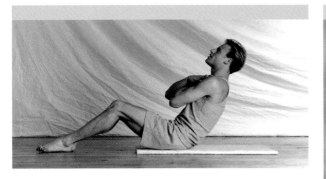

Body lowering

Sit on the floor with your knees slightly bent and pointing up to the ceiling, and cross your hands on your chest. Slowly lower your upper body to the floor for a count of 10, keeping your back straight. Try to keep the movement slow and even. As you become stronger you will be able to take 15 or even 20 seconds to lower your upper body to the ground.

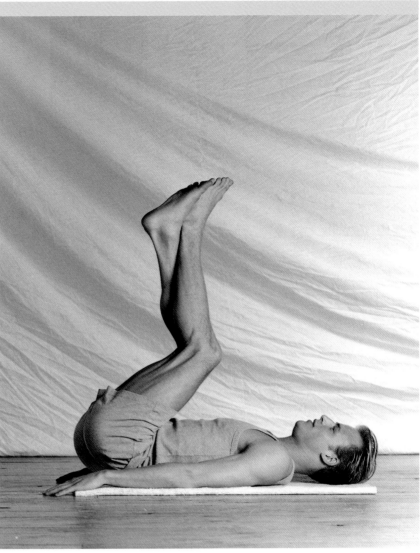

Reverse curl

Lying on your back with knees bent, ankles crossed, and feet flat, tighten your low abdominal muscles and, keeping your back in a natural position, neither arched nor flattened, breathe in and bring your knees slowly up toward your chest. Hold for a few seconds then slowly uncurl as you breathe out, until your feet rest on the floor.

You may do this exercise up to 15 times. The aim is to work on your lower stomach muscles.

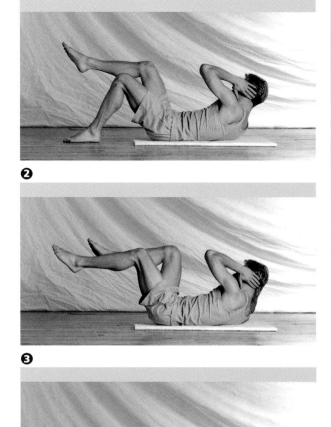

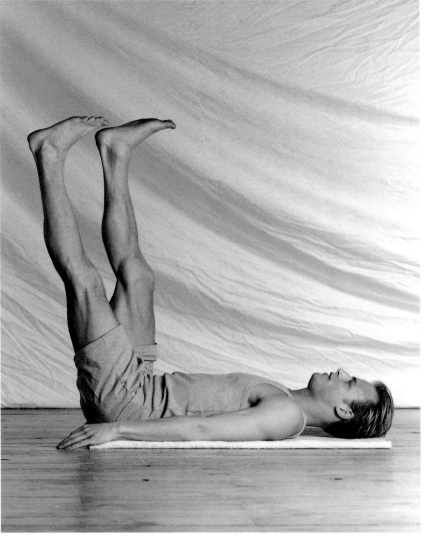

Sprinter

This is an advanced exercise, and you should be very careful to move slowly, smoothly, and with control.

Lying on your back with your knees bent and your hands resting by your ears, lift your right leg so your thigh is vertical. Moving up into the crunch position, twist your upper body so your left elbow moves toward your right knee, and at the same time move your right knee toward your left elbow (1). Relax to the floor, before switching sides. When you are strong enough, you can do the same movement, keeping both legs off the floor (2), or try extending the left leg as you reach toward the right knee with the left elbow (3). Remember to do the same number of repetitions on both sides.

Back walk

Lie on your back on the floor, with your legs straight up in the air and feet flexed. Move your legs back and forth from the hips, as if you were taking very small steps, keeping your feet flexed. Continue for 30 seconds, then bend your knees before lowering your legs back on the floor and relaxing.

Total body workout

For your body to move efficiently, it must have a strong and stable base for the limbs. When a runner gets tired, the trunk and pelvis muscles fatigue first, putting more stress on the back and legs. Similarly, an office worker who sits at a desk all day will also find that trunk and pelvis muscles weaken. This may cause stress on the spine and on the nerves from the neck to the arms, resulting in neck pain and headache.

These exercises increase the stability of your trunk and pelvis by working the muscles of the lower back, the stomach, and the buttocks. You will develop greater awareness of how your trunk and pelvis move and relate to the movements of your arms and legs.

Each day, take a few minutes to do three or four exercises from the torso group and one or two from the buttocks and pelvis and abdominal groups.

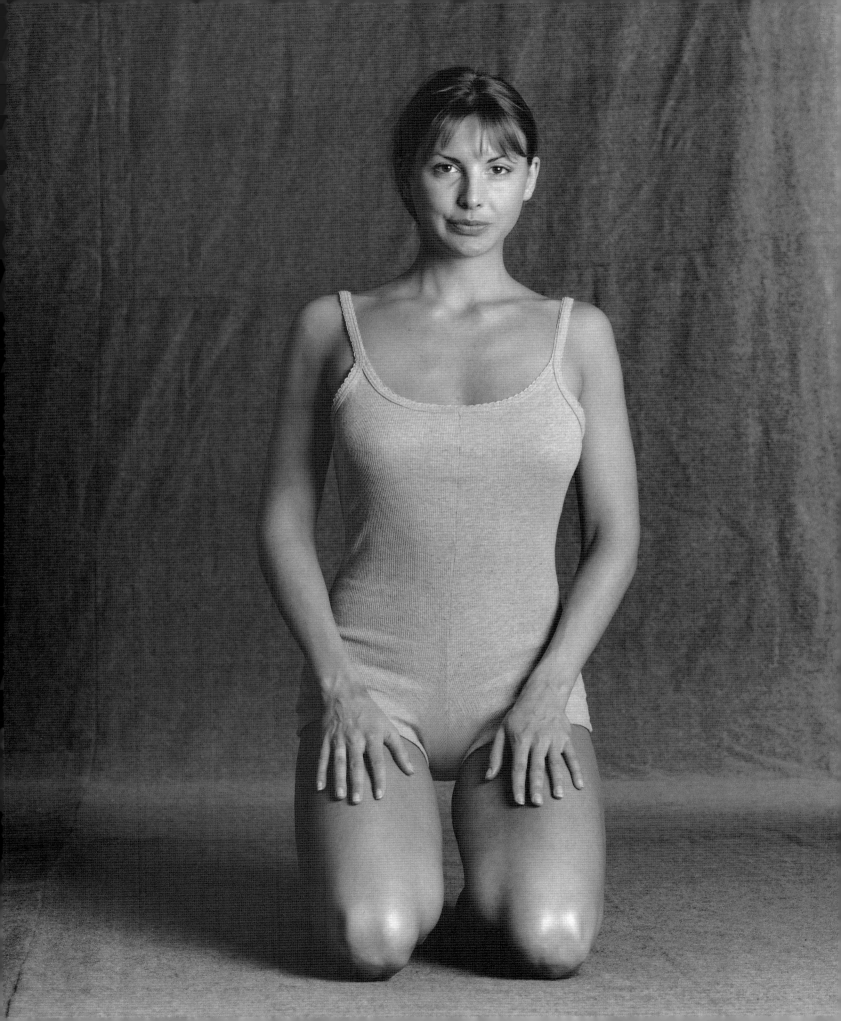

Torso

Your torso – your abdominals, back, chest, and shoulders – is the basis around which your limbs move and is your center of gravity and balance. Therefore, in order to move effectively and efficiently, you must develop the strength and the stability of your torso. The exercises in this section help to enhance the strength and flexibility of the different muscle groups in your trunk, and to improve ways in which these various muscles work intricately together.

❶

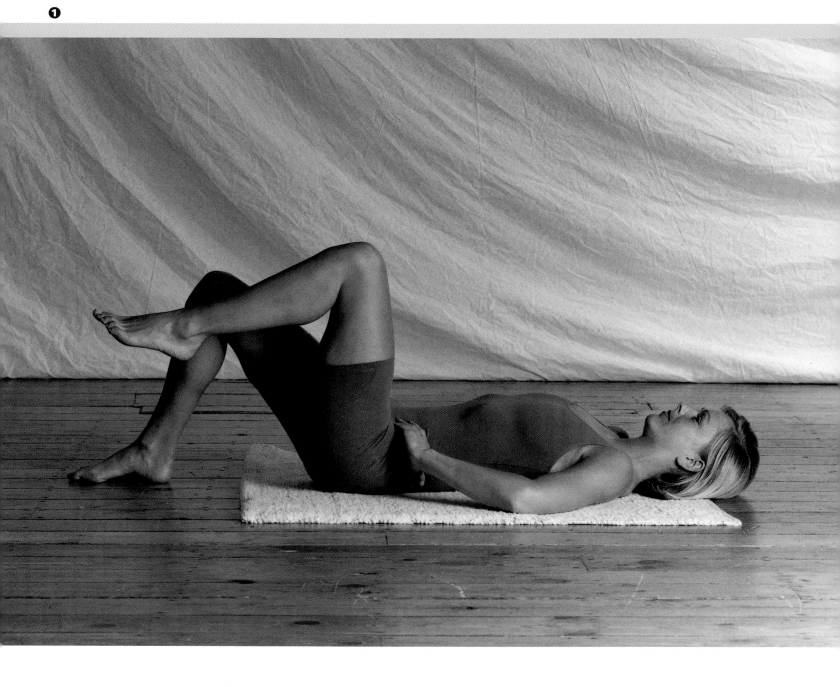

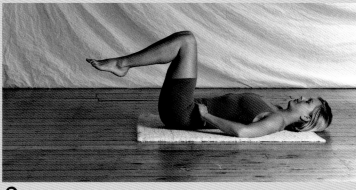

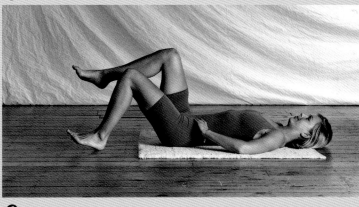

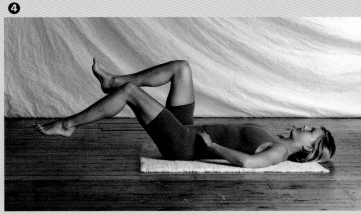

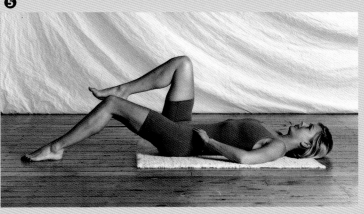

Lying knee lifts

Lie flat on your back with knees bent, your feet and knees in line with your hips, and your feet flat on the floor. It is important that you keep your back straight when you do this, and that there is no movement in your upper body.

1. Lift up your left leg, so your knee is above your hip. Hold this position for 10 seconds, then slowly lower your left leg to the starting position, before switching to the right leg. Repeat this 10 times on each leg. This exercise works the hip flexors and low abdominal muscles.

2. Lift your left leg so your knee is above your hip, and keep your left leg in this position as you lift your right leg to join it.

3. Keeping both your legs in this position and your trunk stable, lower your left leg slowly until your heel touches the floor. Raise your left leg before repeating with the right leg. Repeat 10 times on each leg. This exercise works to strengthen your low abdominal muscles and lower back muscles.

4. This variation should only be done by people with no back pain and who play sport at some level – gymnasts do this exercise regularly. Starting with both your knees above your hips and your back straight and stable, lower your left leg first, but don't let it touch the ground. Keep it slightly off the ground as you slide it out, again making sure that your foot, knee, and hips stay in line and your back remains still. Repeat this exercise six times only on each leg. If you experience any back pain at all, stop right away.

5. Starting with both your knees above your hips and your back stable, slowly lower your left leg so your left foot touches the floor, and, keeping your left foot in contact with the floor, allow your leg to slide down until it is not quite straight. Keep your foot, knee, and hip in line, and do not allow your leg to roll inward. Slowly slide your foot back toward your body and lift your foot so your knee is again above your hip. Repeat on the right leg. Do this exercise 10 times on each side.

1

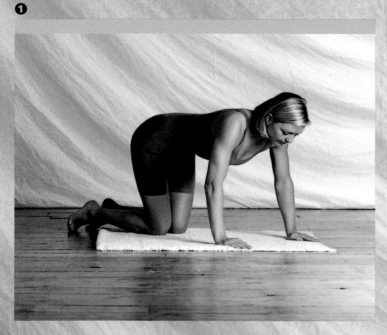

The crawler

Kneel on your hands and knees with your hands under your shoulders, your knees in line with your hips, and your spine straight. The movement is subtle: you should push through your arms to keep your chest raised from the floor (1). Make sure your head is facing forward and not flopped down toward the floor. Hold this position for 15 seconds, and repeat five times.

This exercise works the muscles around your shoulder blades that help to keep your shoulders and neck in a good position. You should not feel any neck or arm pain while you are doing this. If you do, try to work a little more gently, but make sure you stop if the pain persists.

As an advanced variation, you can move your body weight in a diagonal so your weight presses more over the your left hand and your right knee (2). Hold this position for six seconds, then repeat on the other diagonal. Do this exercise at least six times on each side. If you are right-handed, then you should focus on doing two or three more exercises to the right side, and if you are left-handed, you should work a little more to the left.

2

①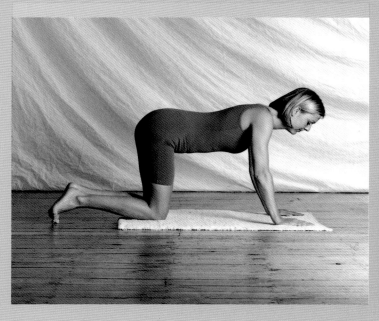

②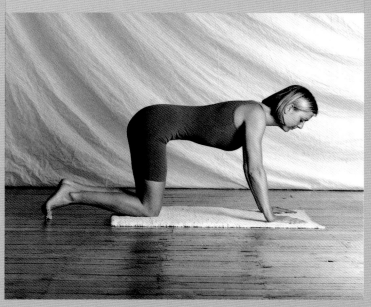

Tummy tuck

Begin on your hands and knees, with your hands in line with your shoulders, your knees in line with your hips, and your spine straight. Keep your head facing forward.

Allow your abdominals to relax so your belly flops down toward the floor (1). Keeping your spine stable, breathe in, allowing your breath to reach all the way down to your stomach. As you breathe out, squeeze your pelvic floor muscles and hollow your low abdominal muscles (2). Do not suck in your whole stomach – the only part of your stomach that should move is the very low part next to your pelvis. As you hold your low stomach hollowed, keep breathing easily. Hold for 20 seconds, relax, and repeat 10 to 12 times.

Bent knee fall-out

Lie on your back, with your hands resting lightly on your hipbones, your knees bent and your feet flat on the floor. As you breathe out, let your left leg gently fall away from your body, but make sure your hips remain still – your hands will feel any movement. Hold for a few seconds, before breathing in and returning your leg to the starting position. Repeat 10 times on each leg.

Buttocks and pelvis

The buttock muscles coordinate the movement of your trunk, and your hips and legs. Parts of the buttock muscles are responsible for twisting the hip and leg outward, and others are responsible for moving your hip and leg backward. The muscles of your low abdomen work with the buttock muscles to stabilize the hips and trunk. These exercises will improve the stability of your pelvic region, strengthen the buttocks and improve their appearance, and will increase mobility in your hips.

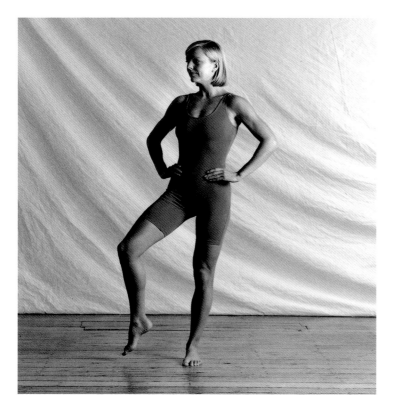

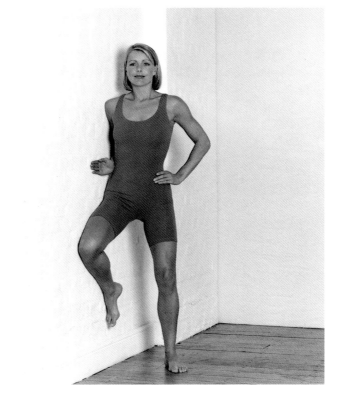

Turnaway

This exercise is slightly more difficult than the side buttock lift (opposite), which uses the same muscles, since it requires additional balance and coordination – but because you work against the force of gravity, it is more dynamic.

Stand with your weight on your left leg, with the knee slightly bent. Lift your right leg off the floor, and keeping your kneecap and foot facing straight ahead, turn your body to the right by pivoting on the left hip. Squeeze your left buttock as you do this movement. Hold this position for 10 seconds before relaxing and repeating six times on each side.

Get it together

This exercise is still more complex and requires a fair degree of trunk and pelvis stability. Stand with your right side to the wall and your right leg bent at the hip and knee. Push the right leg against the wall, and take all of your weight on the left leg.

Bend slightly at the left knee and make sure that your pelvis is facing straight ahead. Squeeze your left buttock and twist out from the left knee and hip. Keep your trunk and pelvis still. Hold this position for 20 seconds, before relaxing and repeating three times on each side. If you feel a twist in your trunk and pelvis, or if you feel unbalanced doing this exercise, go back to the easier exercises in this section for two weeks more before trying again.

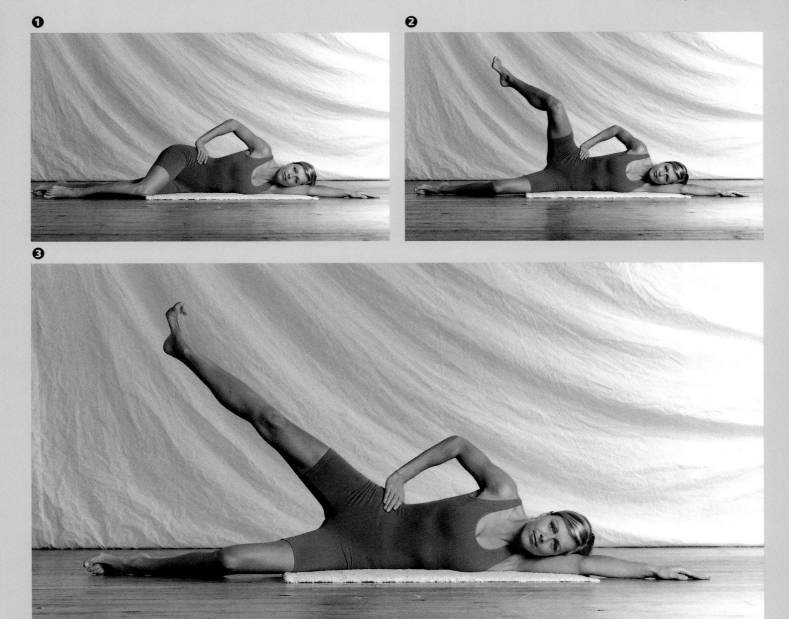

Side buttock lift

This exercise will work the muscles of your buttocks that are responsible for twisting your hip out.

Lying on your side with your bottom leg straight and top leg bent so your knee is almost level with your hip (1), tighten your low abdominal muscles, keeping your back straight. Slowly lift your top knee toward the ceiling, making sure your knee stays bent at the original angle and your trunk does not twist (2). Hold this position for six seconds, then relax. Repeat this exercise six times on each side.

You can vary this exercise by keeping your bottom knee bent and your top leg straight. As you lift your leg toward the ceiling, twist your foot out (3). Hold your leg up for six seconds before lowering it, relaxing, and repeating six times on each leg. Again, make sure your trunk does not twist.

Swimmer

Lying on your stomach with your head turned to one side, tighten your abdominals and your buttock muscles. Keeping both knees straight, raise one leg from the floor, lifting from the hip. Your foot should be no more than four inches (10 cm) from the floor. Do not compensate for the lift by pressing your upper body into the floor – all the movement should come from your hip and pelvis. Hold for 20 seconds before relaxing and repeating on the other leg.

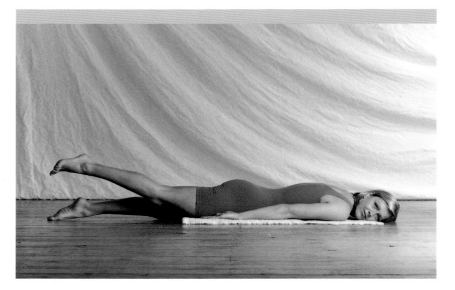

Hip hitch

Lying face down, bend your right knee so your foot is above your knee, gently hollow your low abdominal muscles, and squeeze your buttocks tight. Lift your right knee slightly off the floor, moving from your hip. Hold this position for 10 seconds before relaxing, and repeat 10 times on each side.

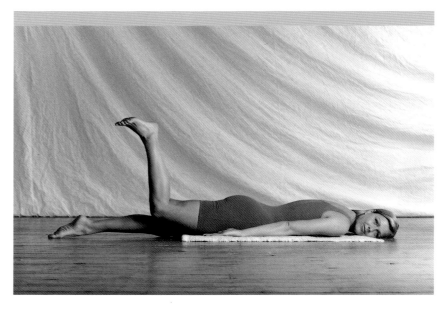

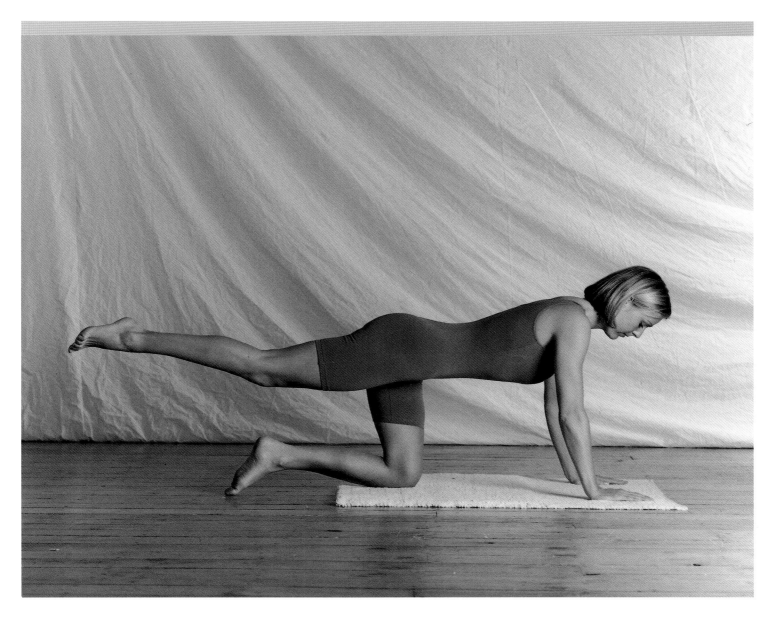

Kickback

This exercise works your abdominal and back muscles at the same time as it tones your buttock muscles.

On your hands and knees, tighten your lower abdominal muscles and keep your back straight and relaxed. Straighten your right knee and hip to raise your leg straight behind you as if kicking backward. Maintain this position for three seconds, before relaxing and repeating six times on each leg. It is important to keep the rest of your body as stable as possible as you kick back with your moving leg.

As an advanced variation, you can reach up with your left arm at the same time as you reach back with your left leg. Again, hold for three seconds, and repeat six times on each leg.

Abdominals

The abdominals are the muscles running from the ribs down to the pelvis, and also from the spinal vertebrae of the lower back around to the front of the stomach. These muscles bend the trunk forward and maintain stability of the trunk in conjunction with the lower back muscles. If these muscles are flabby and weak, it is not only unattractive – you also risk suffering from lower back pain, because the muscles are not supporting your trunk. You should choose two or three exercises to do from this section. They are some of the most important exercises to include in your daily practice.

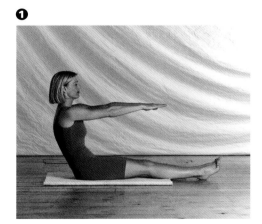

❶ ❷ ❸

Toe reach

Lying flat on your back with your legs out straight, tighten your low abdominal muscles, and slowly curl up: drop your chin toward your chest, then curl from the top of your chest, reaching toward your toes (1). When you are sitting up, tighten your low abdominals again and slowly uncurl until you are lying flat. You can also vary the arm position to make the exercise more challenging, either crossing your arms across your chest (2), or placing your hands lightly against your temples (3).

Do not try this exercise if you get any lower back pain. At first, do not do too many repetitions. If your legs start to lift from the floor, it is a sure sign that you have done too much and your abdominals have fatigued. Breathe deeply to relax.

The crunch

Lying on your back with your hips and knees bent to right angles and your lower legs and feet resting on a sofa or chair, tighten your low abdominal muscles and keep your lower back stable. With arms folded across your chest or with your hands placed lightly against your temples, curl up slowly, head and upper back first, until you reach your limit. Hold this position for three seconds before slowly lowering your body to the floor.

Repeat this exercise with a slight twist, so that as you come up, your right shoulder moves toward your left knee. Next time, your left shoulder moves toward your right knee.

Repeat a maximum of 15 times, stopping if you get tired.

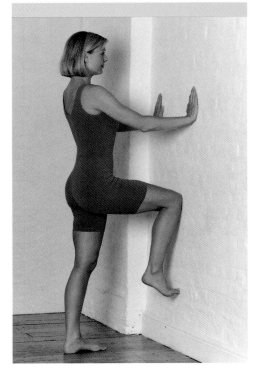

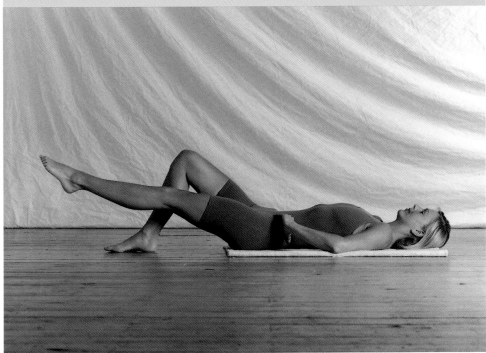

Run-through

Stand facing a wall, with your hands placed on the wall at shoulder level, squeezing your buttock muscles and tightening your low abdominal muscles. Slowly lift your right leg from the hip, keeping your hip, knee, and foot in line, until it is bent at right angles from the hip. Hold this position for 20 seconds. Repeat three times on each leg.

Leg raise

Lying on your back, with your right knee bent and right foot flat on the floor, tighten your lower abdominal muscles and keep your lower back stable, neither arching nor flattening it. With your left knee straight and toes pointing, slowly lift your left leg slightly off the floor. Hold this position for 10 seconds before slowly relaxing and repeating on the other leg. Do this exercise 10 times on each leg.

Seated crease

Sitting in a chair, straighten your back so you lift up your chest, and tighten your low abdominal muscles. Slowly lift your right leg from the hip, bringing your knee slightly toward you and keeping it bent at the same angle. All the movement should come from your right side – don't use your left leg to push, and don't lean to the left. Hold this position for 15 seconds, before relaxing and repeat six times on each leg.

Routines

It is not difficult to fit regular exercise into your day-to-day life, especially when you do not have to devote a long block of time to it. Here are some exercises that take only a few minutes and are tailored for different circumstances.

Pause gymnastics are exercises designed to be done every half-hour when you are working at a desk. They will help you to avoid the stiffness and strain that comes from a sedentary lifestyle.

Home energizers are perfect for people who do not play sports or go to fitness classes, but want to stretch and tone the body through exercises at home.

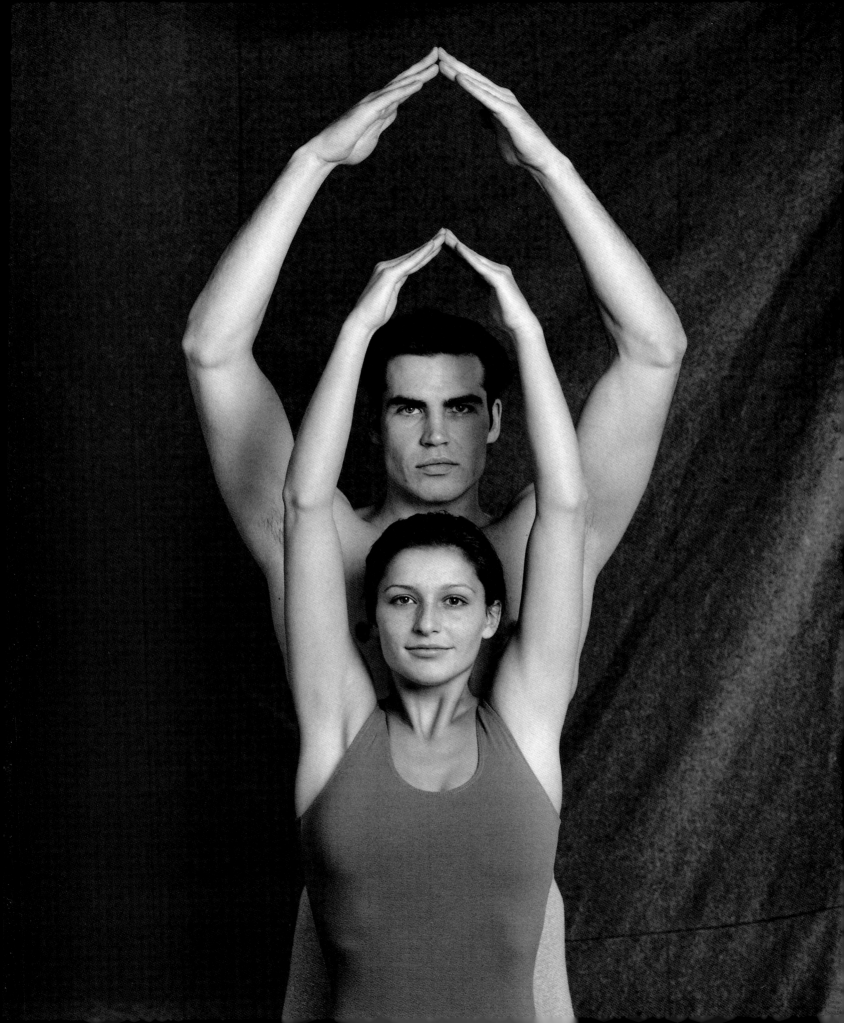

Pause gymnastics

Choose two or three of the following exercises to do every half-hour when you are sitting at a desk or working at a keyboard. They will fend off the stiffness that comes from sitting at a desk all day and will improve your postural awareness. The stretches for your forearms and hands will also keep your wrist joints flexible and the tendons in your forearms and wrists supple. These are familiar problem areas for people who work on keyboards or do repetitive tasks during the day.

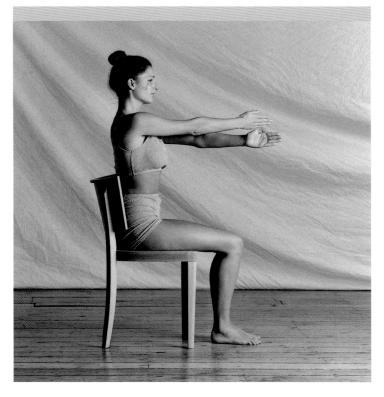

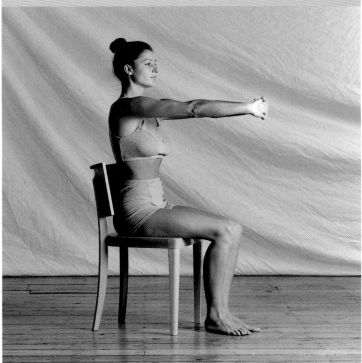

Shoulder stretch

Sit tall, lifting a little at your chest. Reach out in front with both your arms, with your elbows and wrists straight and keeping your shoulder blades tucked back and down. Slowly cross your arms from the shoulders until you feel a stretch in both shoulders.

When you feel the stretch, hold the position for 10 seconds. Relax and repeat three times. This is a good stretch for the muscles at the top of your shoulders, which tend to tighten if you sit at your desk for long periods of time.

Palm pull

This exercise will stretch your wrist and elbow joints as well as the tendons in your forearms. Sit tall, lifting a little at your chest. Reach straight out in front of you from your shoulders, and interlace your fingers so your palms are facing toward you, then turn your palms away at the wrist. Stretch your arms forward from your shoulders. Hold this position for six seconds then relax and repeat twice. Make sure you keep a good upper back position as you do this exercise.

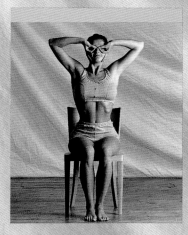

Mr Magoo

This funny position will stretch your upper arms and forearms. Sitting tall and lifting a little at your chest, make circles with the thumb and index finger of both hands. This is the tricky part: turn your palms up and over toward your face, with your fingers pointing down and resting along the side of your face, so the circles you made with your thumb and index finger fit around your eyes like glasses. Lift your elbows to stretch your arms slightly behind you. Hold this stretch for three seconds and repeat three times.

Wrestler hold

Sitting tall and lifting a little at your chest, reach with your right hand around your back and up in between your shoulder blades. Reach as far as you can, feeling a stretch at the front of your shoulder and in between your shoulder blades. Hold this stretch for three seconds before relaxing and repeating three times on each arm.

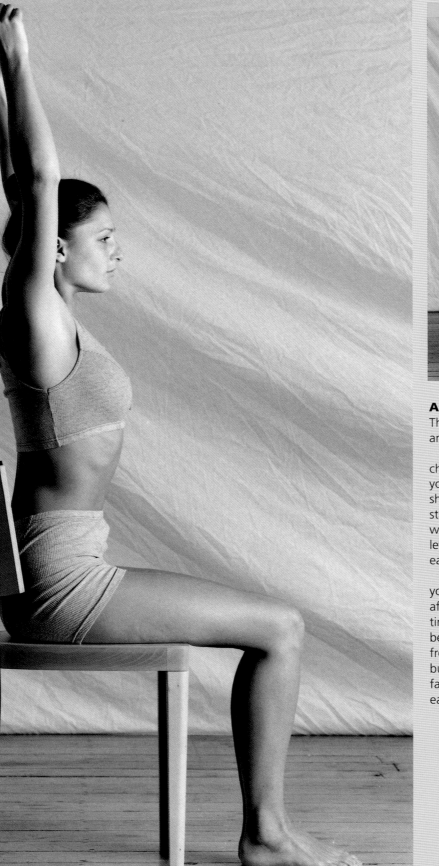

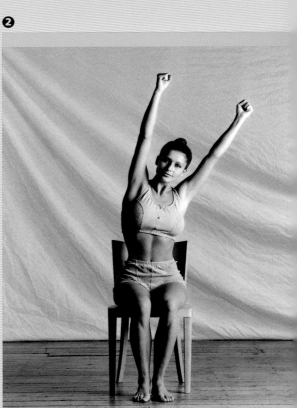

Arm extender

This exercise will loosen your upper back and your arms.

Sitting tall and lifting a little at your chest, make fists and reach with both of your arms above your head (1). Your shoulders, elbows, and hands should be straight above you. Reach a little higher with your right hand, and then with your left. Repeat this exercise three times on each arm.

You can vary this position so it stretches your entire spine – this variation is ideal after you have been sitting for a long time. With your arms straight above you, bend sideways, starting the movement from low down your torso, keeping both buttocks on the chair and your chest facing forward (2). Repeat three times on each side.

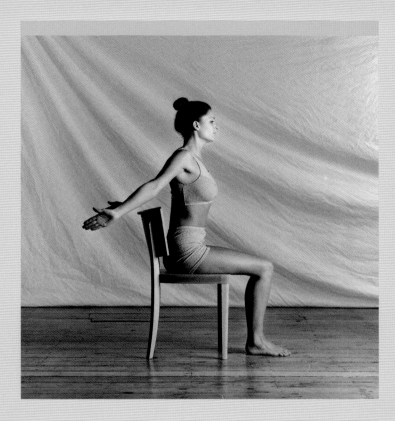

Airplane

Sitting tall, lift a little at your chest and rotate your hands so your palms face the ceiling, your thumbs pointing behind you. Raise your arms, keeping them straight, and draw them gently behind your back. Hold your arms out straight like wings, maintaining the stretch for six seconds. Repeat this exercise three times.

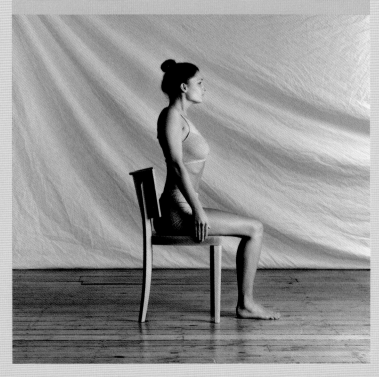

Seated shoulder circle

This exercise will help you to relax your upper back and free your shoulders. Sit tall in your chair, lifting a little at your chest. Shrug your shoulders up toward your ears and then roll them backward, making sure the movement is coming from your shoulders. Repeat this circular movement six times. Relax the shoulder muscles as you let go of each circle.

Home energizers

These exercises are specifically designed for people who do not play sports or participate in any other fitness activities, but who are looking for simple, effective exercises that stretch and tone the whole body. You don't even have to do them all at once.

They take only a few seconds each, so they are can easily be incorporated into your day-to-day life. Try doing a few during the commercial breaks of your favorite TV show or when you take a break from reading or preparing something to eat.

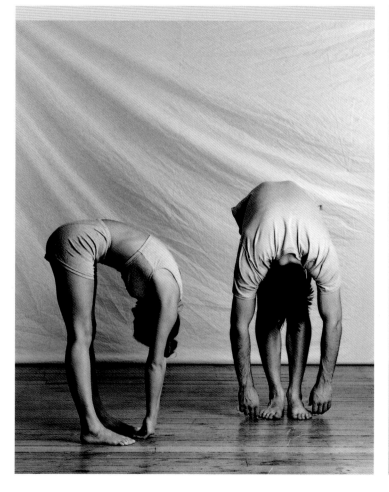

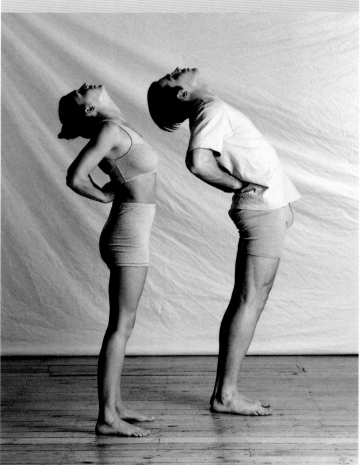

The puppet
Imagine yourself suspended by strings like a puppet. Think how it would feel if the strings supporting the top of your body broke.

Stand with your weight equally over both feet. Starting with your head, curl forward so your chin touches your chest, then continue the curling movement from your upper back down. Relax totally into the stretch for 10 seconds. On the way back up, gently uncurl from your lower back to your upper back, then your neck and head.

Standing cobra
Stand with your weight equally through both of your legs and knees straight but not locked. Make fists with your hands and place them in the small of your back, and tuck your elbows behind you. Keep your head facing to the front as you arch back over your fists. Hold this stretch for six seconds before relaxing and repeating three times. Don't push this stretch too far, especially if you have a weak lower back. When your back is supple, you can include your head in the backward bend.

Simon says

Standing with your weight equally over both feet and your knees straight, place your hands on your head, and without twisting from your waist, bend to the side so your left shoulder moves toward your left hip. Don't push too far – you should feel a gentle stretch in your back. Return to the starting position, then repeat on the other side. Repeat slowly and gently four times on each side.

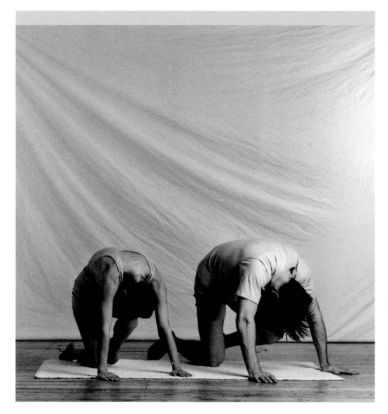

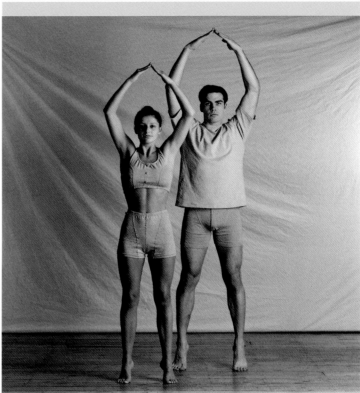

Advanced crawl

Begin on your hands and knees on the floor, with your back and neck straight. Bend your left knee up toward your chest, and as you do, tuck your chin down toward your chest, curling your back. Keep your weight balanced through both of your hands and your right knee.

Repeat this exercise six times on each leg. This will improve the suppleness of your whole spine.

Ballet dancer

This is a good exercise for your upper back, buttocks, and low abdominal muscles.

Standing with your weight on the balls of your feet, raise yourself onto your toes, maintaining your balance. As you breathe in deeply, raise both arms out to the side and up so that your hands touch above your head. Slowly breathe out as you lower yourself onto flat feet and allow your arms to return to your sides. Take your time, concentrating on your balance, and try to reach as high as you can.

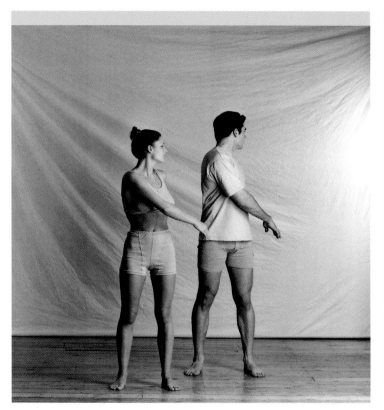

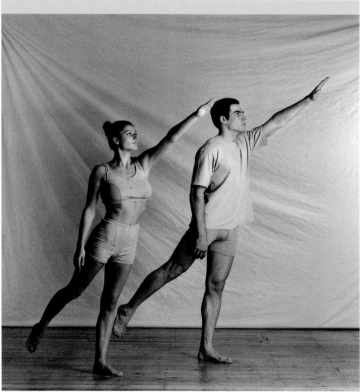

Pinwheel

Stand with your weight equally over both feet and your knees slightly bent. Twist your head, shoulders, and trunk to the left, then return to the starting position before twisting to the other side. Repeat six times on each side. This is a good stretch for your spine, but it also works the muscles of your back, neck, and shoulders.

Diagonal reach

Stand, balancing with most of your weight on your left leg. Concentrating on maintaining your balance, reach forward and up with your left arm and raise your right leg behind you. You can place your left arm lightly on a wall for balance. Repeat this movement three times with your left arm and right leg, then three times for the right arm and left leg.

This exercise will improve the flexibility of your spine, shoulder, and hip joints. It will also tone the muscles of your buttocks, stomach, and upper back.

Index

Acknowledgments

Illustrations: Marks Creative

Additional text: Sara Black

Proofreader: Phyllida Hancock

Indexer: Clare Richards

Chair: Montego, by Habitat

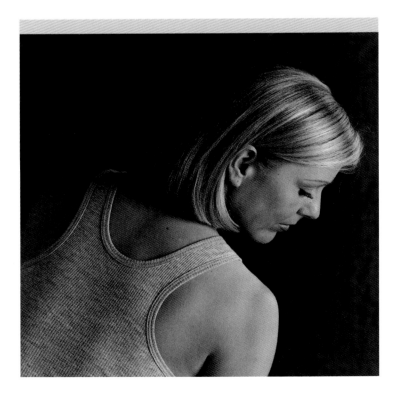